HOLDING SPACE

of related interest

The Yoga Teacher Mentor
A Reflective Guide to Holding Spaces, Maintaining
Boundaries, and Creating Inclusive Classes
Jess Glenny
Foreword by Norman Blair
ISBN 978 1 78775 126 2
eISBN 978 1 78775 127 9

Yoga Student Handbook
Develop Your Knowledge of Yoga Principles and Practice
Edited by Sian O'Neill
Foreword by Lizzie Lasater
ISBN 978 0 85701 386 6
eISBN 978 0 85701 388 0

Yoga Teaching Handbook
A Practical Guide for Yoga Teachers and Trainees
Edited by Sian O'Neill
ISBN 978 1 84819 355 0
eISBN 978 0 85701 313 2

The Guided Meditation Handbook
Advice, Meditation Scripts and Hasta Mudra for Yoga Teachers
Georgia Keal
ISBN 978 1 78775 048 7
eISBN 978 1 78775 049 4

Restoring Prana
A Therapeutic Guide to Pranayama and Healing Through the Breath
for Yoga Therapists, Yoga Teachers, and Healthcare Practitioners
Robin L. Rothenberg
Foreword by Richard Miller
Illustrated by Kirsteen Wright
ISBN 978 1 84819 401 4
eISBN 978 0 85701 357 6

HOLDING SPACE

The Creative Performance and
Voice Workbook for Yoga Teachers

SARAH SCHARF, MFA

Foreword by Judith Hanson Lasater, Ph.D., P.T.

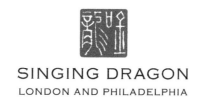

SINGING DRAGON

LONDON AND PHILADELPHIA

First published in Great Britain in 2021 by Singing
Dragon, an imprint of Jessica Kingsley Publishers
An Hachette Company

1

The epigraph on page 61 is reproduced with kind permission from
Kristin Linklater Voice Centre. The voice and diction evaluation form on
page 95 is reproduced from Anderson (1997) *Training the Speaking Voice*
with permission of Oxford Publishing Limited through PLSclear.

A CIP catalogue record for this title is available from the
British Library and the Library of Congress

ISBN 978 1 84819 405 2
eISBN 978 0 85701 361 3

Printed and bound by CPI Group (UK) Ltd, Croydon, CR0 4YY

Jessica Kingsley Publishers' policy is to use papers that are natural,
renewable and recyclable products and made from wood grown in
sustainable forests. The logging and manufacturing processes are expected
to conform to the environmental regulations of the country of origin.

Jessica Kingsley Publishers
73 Collier Street
London N1 9BE, UK

www.singingdragon.com

To my grandmothers, Rose and Helen, who would have loved to tell their friends that I wrote a book; and to my son, Jasper, who I hope will value his accomplishments through the lens of his own heart.

Acknowledgements

I could not have written this book without the help and input from so many.

I thank my husband for all the times he supported me as I struggled to complete this project.

With gratitude I appreciate the countless lessons I have learned from all of the students I have had the privilege to teach.

A massive thank you to my main yoga teacher, Judith Hanson Lasater, who honestly gave advice on the task of book writing and continues to be a beacon for me of graceful and purposeful living.

To Elizabeth Stanley and all the staff at the Life Centre and Yogacampus in London for the chance to grow and be nurtured by a remarkable organization.

To Claire Wilson for asking me if I was interested in turning my workshop into a book!

To Rosalia Aloguin Dols for her artistic talent and friendship.

To Rychel Scott for her photos and encouragement.

To Philipp Dunbar for his modelling skills and studentship.

To Adam Hocke for his words and his ability to call when I most need a friend.

To Bridget Luff for her writing and friendship.

To Lizzie Lasater for her generosity and writing.

To David Kim for the opportunity to learn and lending his thoughts.

To Thea Maillard for the lovely yoga nidrā script and for being my neighbor.

To Giulia Tamiazzo for the beautiful space she created at Retreat in Vienna.

To Michael Morgan for his quick replies and help in tracking down texts and for introducing me to voice work at UCSB, and all the faculty of the Drama Department.

To Jim Libby for his improv inspiration and recommendations.

To all of my colleagues and teachers from London International School of Performing Arts. I am so lucky to have you and the Lecoq pedagogy experience in my life keeping me sane and my laughter flowing.

To all of my friends and family who listened as I went through this birth process of making the book.

To Kristin Linklater, who passed away during the writing of this book: may her memory be a blessing.

Lastly, to my parents and my sister who know how truly dramatic I can be and still love me.

Contents

Foreword

Teaching yoga is not just about what you know. It is actually more about how well you are able to *communicate* what you know, so that the student takes in your words and understands them deeply in his or her own body and mind.

Sarah Scharf has written a comprehensive book to help us all investigate how to do this. In *Holding Space* she has taken us on a step-by-step investigation into how the words, tone, volume, as well as the intention of our speech, meld together to create communication.

She also offers us some asana practice and self-reflective suggestions and exercises that help us to prepare the vessel from which our voice emanates.

Sarah is in a unique position to write such a book. She has an extensive background in both yoga and theater, both of which are first and foremost about communicating. I first met her in my yoga class, and to say she was enthusiastic and curious about the restorative yoga I was teaching is an understatement.

She soon started showing up in my workshops at various places around the world, and we gradually became colleagues, and finally friends as well. Her bright demeanor and infectious laugh have made her easy to work with over the years as she began to assist me.

I am grateful to her for this book. Teaching is primarily a relationship: first we need to have a clear relationship with ourselves. And then we are better prepared to have a healthy relationship with our students. The basis of all relationships is, of course, the ability and willingness to communicate. Most yoga teacher training programs with which I am familiar teach their trainees *what to say*, but not how to *communicate*. Sarah teaches us the difference, and opens our eyes and ears to how we might improve our skills to allow for complete communication. She teaches us this in a way that is integrated and clear.

Thank you, Sarah, for your passion for learning, and as well for your dedication to helping us all to be the best teachers we can be by offering us this book.

> *Judith Hanson Lasater*, Ph.D., P.T., cofounder of *Yoga Journal* and
> The California Yoga Teachers Association, author and master teacher

INTRODUCTION

For every existing yoga teacher, there are two more yoga teachers currently in training.[1] As yoga grows in popularity so does the need for quality teaching. No matter what style of yoga you teach, chances are your training focused on the practices, anatomy and practicalities of starting to work. Most teacher trainings today are a standard 200-hour model, which is only enough time to introduce how to safely teach group classes and understand the how and why of what you teach. It's possible to touch on the importance of using your voice and presence to teach. Maybe some time is spent on how to create an environment in your classes that promotes inclusion, welcoming and authenticity. Rarely, however, is time spent on this topic in a thorough way that actually leaves you with a strong skill set. Many trainings end with a practice teaching session, after which you will be lucky to receive feedback on your teaching. This might be the only time you get this kind of constructive criticism from experts helping you grow as a teacher. Most feedback for new teachers includes improving the voice, dealing with nerves and connecting more with the group of people being taught. Then new graduates are sent off to figure out how to do that on their own.

Many teachers hear this feedback and then find few options on learning how to actually make it happen. Searching online or in guidebooks for yoga teacher improvement, I found more of the same—instructions to speak loudly enough for the students in the back to hear you, with no tools on how to safely make that happen. In my research I also saw many notes on avoiding a "yoga teacher voice" but again nothing on what steps to take, or even what a yoga teacher voice is! This book is a guide to effective voice work and stage presence for yoga teachers.

Wherever you are in your path as a teacher, working on your voice and presence will make you a better teacher. It is another element of yourself to explore and build awareness. The better you know your own voice and your comfort level with speaking to large groups, the better you can teach and expand your edges.

Voice work is its own practice. Just as a yoga practice grows day by day, learning to improve your voice and presence as the teacher grows one step at a time. When we approach a complex yoga posture, we know it will take time to develop the component parts of breath, physical ability and mental focus. To an inexperienced yogi these poses can seem overwhelming or mysterious. It is the same with voice and presence—we must understand the component parts of how best to use our voices and be present as the teacher. It is not a mystery and it is not a gift from birth. It is a skill that can be learned and practiced. This book will teach you how.

WHY THIS BOOK?

I was a performer from a young age. I loved being the center of attention and spent most of my time making up plays and dances, rehearsing physical gestures endlessly to get it just right. My mother was a schoolteacher and a singer. She has a rich singing voice and a speaking voice that commanded attention. As much as I loved performing, I was told early on that my singing voice was not so good and I always thought of my other family members as the musical ones, constantly comparing my voice with my mother's. It never seemed to measure up.

As a speaker I had many opportunities to grow. I remember winning a poetry competition and reading my poem at the governor's office when I was eight years old, school theater productions and acting classes where I worked on being heard. I remember my Bat Mitzvah, singing and leading the Saturday morning prayer service and delivering a speech at 13 to over one hundred people. By 17 I was teaching theater and dance to children, where I learned quickly to use my voice to keep the room in control and the kids from going wild. Looking back at my childhood, I see the story of my voice and how I learned to be comfortable in front of an audience, as myself not just as an actor.

Studying acting, directing and playwriting, I continued to learn the tools I use today as a yoga teacher. When I began to train as a yoga teacher and eventually teach I was lucky to have a background that gave me a platform to teach from. I continue to be inspired by my work in theater to explore the essence of communication and the complexity of human nature. This informs my yoga teaching and allows me to work like a director to mentor and help teachers develop their own power and confidence in vocal work. Coaching teachers on how best to use their voices and helping them recognize their own vocal histories is a joy and an honor for me. I want to elevate the standard of teaching in the yoga world and help teachers develop their potential to speak in an embodied way that connects the philosophy of yoga to the act of standing in front of a room of students and saying clearly, "Let's begin."

HOW I FOUND YOGA

When I was 19 I trained to become a massage therapist. As a freshman at university my back had spasmed from stress and my first professional massage was a life-changing experience. Imagining all the people I could help, I also thought it would be a good side job while I tried to find work as an actress. At that time I had never heard of Reiki, practiced yoga only sporadically and was intent on pursuing an Academy Award. I spent a lot of my time going to parties and focusing on my social life, which was of course very dramatic. Learning about anatomy and studying the human body was fascinating and I happily aced my massage certification exams. To complete the diploma required me to work more than 50 hours in the student clinic, which gave discounted massages to the community as a way of training the graduates. During my course with fellow trainees and working on friends to practice the techniques had been very easy for me. When the time came to work with the public, I was not prepared for the myriad of emotions that came up. At one point I started a session by placing my hands slowly on the client's back, which was covered by a cotton sheet. When my hands made contact with their back, I felt a wave of heat travel up my arms and I began to cry quite intensely. I had never experienced anything like this before and it scared me. I excused myself and got one of the teachers who was supervising the clinic to step in for me. After the client left my teacher suggested that I practice Reiki, a healing technique based on the Japanese theory of channeling universal energy. She recommended that I use Reiki to help me keep my energetic boundaries fortified and explained what an empath is. I was so overwhelmed by this experience and daunted by the idea that I would need to change my partying lifestyle that I quit the clinic and with only four hours left to complete my certification I gave up.

Four years later, after burning out on partying, I found myself planning my life around my yoga classes. Soon after, I traveled through Costa Rica on my own and in the rainforest along the Pacuare River I decided to become a yoga teacher. When I returned to California, I enrolled in the first of many yoga teacher trainings and stepped onto the path that has led me to where I sit writing this book. This initial training was with Ana Forrest in Los Angeles. Many people on the training have personal breakthroughs and breakdowns due to the intense nature of the work, so there was a requirement to have a therapist on deck. As a child and also as a teenager I had done some counseling to help deal with my parents' divorce. At the time I felt quite content and didn't think I needed to be in therapy. I found a therapist who specialized in growth therapy and the connection between body and mind. Her business card read "the issues are in our tissues," which struck me as totally true. Thanks to the combination of yoga and therapy I came to understand my empathic nature and accept it. My practice began to help me find my energetic boundaries and the space within to be present with other people's difficult emotions. I went back to the massage clinic and completed my hours, after which I trained further in massage therapy at the Esalen Institute and began to work with yoga students, combining massage and restorative yoga. As I have found my niche in training other teachers, the work I do to keep clear energetic boundaries continues to be a vital part of how I work. I see the practice of yoga as one part of my spiritual practice, and an anchor that helps me to teach and fulfill my dharma.

HOW TO USE THIS BOOK

I have written this book as a a guide and workbook, something to come back to at different stages in your life as a teacher and speaker. I encourage you to take your time, to linger with the questions to give your mind time to process new ideas, and your heart time to process the emotional work.

As part of your voice training, try recording yourself reading instructions for the exercises so that you can do them without looking at the book. This will help you get more comfortable with your own voice and help you to improve your sense of timing when you are teaching others.

The first chapters will introduce you to your own voice and the process of voice work, both physical and emotional. Starting with yoga practices you might already know to ease you into the different type of practice that is working with your voice.

Chapter 3 deals with communication and Chapter 4 with physical theater and improvisation techniques to help you respond to the moment. Chapter 5 is a groundwork to see how you set the stage for your classes and find the most supportive way to teach.

In Chapter 6 we will look closely at how different people learn, so that when you teach you have more understanding of different learners.

Pro Tips are aimed at teachers who are holding workshops, trainings, intensives and retreats that require teaching for multiple hours and often travel.

Chapters 7 and 8 go into curriculum planning and themes that are important considerations at this level of teaching. Just as we never get beyond needing to practice, if we want to sustain long teaching hours we need to maintain our vocal practice and make sure we are warming up our voices for teaching.

The last chapter will help you to source mentorship and further study as well as giving more tools to help you find inspiration.

Sections marked "Pro tip" are aimed at teachers who are holding workshops, trainings, intensives and retreats that require teaching for multiple hours and often travel.

For now, as you begin this journey of mapping and expanding your voice as a teacher, I leave you with a quote to help navigate your own personal learning process with this book:

It takes over **400** repetitions to create a synapse in the brain (true learning) <u>without</u> playful engagement or about **12** repetitions to create a synapse when you use play to teach. So, if you really want to effectively and efficiently teach your children (or anyone for that matter), use PLAY! (Dr. Karyn Purvis[2])

PRECAUTIONS FOR PRACTICE

Take caution when starting to practice new poses and exercises. During pregnancy and menstruation avoid inversions and take extra care not to stretch to your full range of movement. For pregnancy avoid all pressure on the abdomen and twists that compress the front of the body. If you have any disc disorders or injuries to the spine please use twists, forward folds and backbends with only half of your possible range of movement, wait a day and see if you can progress slowly towards deeper poses. Anyone with serious injuries or health conditions should consult a physician and practice with care at their own liability.

Whenever possible learning from a teacher that can give you direct feedback is best. I look forward to meeting you online or in person at one of my teaching events or for individual coaching and mentoring; do not hesitate to reach out.

www.sarahscharf.com

ANATOMY OF THE VOICE

START AT THE VERY BEGINNING

The beauty of beginning a voice practice is that it can be done on its own or within the context of your existing personal yoga practice. If you don't yet have a home practice, this might help you start one (wink, wink). Learning to instinctively follow your own physical impulses will help you on your journey to expressing yourself as a teacher. Many of the prānāyāma or breathing techniques you might already know will be perfect tools to help develop your voice. As with any new practice, the ground of the work is what you start with.

GOING INWARD: YOUR HISTORY

Most of us have some scars concerning our attitude toward our voices. In many ways the voice can be closely linked with our identity. Acknowledging your emotional relationship to your voice is an important step in this process. If you uncover difficult emotions, please reach out for support from anyone that is a fan of *you*. Remember, you need a positive cheerleader, not another critic! On that note, remember to be gentle with yourself. Take some time to journal or meditate on the following questions.

What do you like about your voice?

_____

_____

_____

How do you feel about your voice? Do you enjoy hearing recordings of yourself?

_____

_____

_____

What are your first memories of speaking?

_____

_____

_____

Can you remember a time when you were praised or shamed for speaking up? Allow yourself to stay with the memories and the feelings.

_____

_____

_____

Have you had positive or negative feedback about the quality of your voice? Who gave you this feedback? Was it constructive? How did you receive the feedback?

_____

_____

_____

_____

_____

We all have a unique history that makes us who we are. It is the same for the voice. Just as we see physical patterns of tension in our yoga work, the voice has patterns of use or misuse. The measured parts of your individual voice are called a voiceprint. Just like a fingerprint, no two voiceprints are the same. Your voiceprint is like a picture of the way that you sound. Our speech, the rhythm that we speak with, the use of inflection and intonation are influenced by where you grew up and learned to speak. For example, people who grow up in large cities tend to speak faster, and have accents that are clipped and more staccato in rhythm. People who grow up in slower-paced places tend to speak more slowly and have a more musical cadence. Start to listen to the people around you, maybe to the teachers you admire, with an ear for the qualities of the voices you enjoy. Another element in the speed we speak with is the rate of our thoughts. Sometimes people think faster than they can speak, which tends to make us trip over our words or stutter.

As you begin this process, what will help the most is cultivating a playful and non-judgmental attitude. The next element in your voice practice is to have compassion for yourself. In essence, the vocal practice is another form of mindfulness. The more attention and focus you bring to this learning process, the more you will feel deep improvement.

Before you begin your vocal journey, take some time to give yourself empathy and practice self-compassion. I recommend you create an intention, or san kalpa (Sanskrit) for your voice work. Intentions are different from goals. They do not place the focus on outcome, but rather on the quality of the process. Having a san kalpa is very helpful during your practice to help you feel your limits and work safely. Simply wanting to be better at something creates layers of tension within us. Set an intention in your own words that encompasses staying present with how you feel and staying open to growth. Perhaps this includes an image that represents growth and expansion. Maybe for you a certain color, music or even scent will help you in finding your intention.

GUIDED MEDITATION

This is a meditation based on mindful body scanning to help you set your intention.

Sit or lie in a comfortable position, in a safe place where you will be undisturbed. Read each line of this meditation and then pause to feel and notice as instructed.

Adjust your physical position to be even more comfortable. What areas of your body are you able to relax more? Relax them. Bring attention to your breath without changing it. Notice the quality and texture of your breath. Allow it to be just as it is. Notice the sensations in your abdomen. Let any tension you feel there go. Allow it to be enough. Accept what you feel. Relax your jaw so that your teeth release from pressing together. Let the lips part softly. Allow your tongue to feel heavy and thick. Notice your breathing. Feel the area of your chest. Let the ribs move freely. Notice how the ribs move. Be aware of the inner throat. Let the throat feel wider and softer. Any uncomfortable sensations or emotions are OK. Notice them and allow yourself to stay connected to feeling them as you let go of any arising thoughts. Any pleasurable feelings are OK. Notice them and allow yourself to stay connected to feeling as you let go of any arising thoughts. In your own words set an intention to be kind to yourself, to have more compassion and empathy for any struggles or judgment that will come up during your practice. Breathe smoothly as you repeat this intention three times silently. Repeat your intention out loud. Inhale the breath. Press each fingertip firmly against your thumb, one by one. See clearly the place that you are in. Feel your feet; press them against the ground.

Take a moment now to write some notes here about your experience and record your intention. Each time you practice you can set a new intention or continue with this one if it still feels meaningful. Having this to look back on as you work will be a tangible way to keep track of your progress. Remember that progress looks more like this

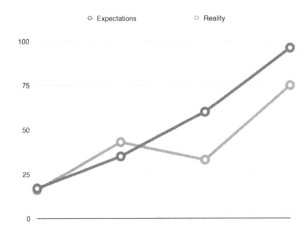

Or something even more like a wave, with movement in the back and forth realm more than we often allow for. Enjoy the ride!

_____

_____

_____

_____

_____

THE INSTRUMENT

We make sound every day, yet most of us don't know much about how. The human voice is an amazing instrument. We are wind instruments and our awareness of this is the first step in learning how to play well. The main parts of our instrument are briefly defined here. This chapter continues with yogic practices to begin getting to know and then strengthening your instrument.

Lungs

Our lungs pump the air and control the pressure over the vocal folds, which makes them vibrate. The vibration is what creates sound. Human lungs expand most noticeably in the lower segments and towards the back of the body. This is why the work of the diaphragm is essential to good lung function. Tension or dysfunction in the diaphragm will stop the lungs from being able to fully expand, causing a shorter breath. We experience this when we are stressed or emotional; in extreme cases like panic attacks people feel unable to breathe at all. A shorter, more shallow breath leads to less power for creating, sustaining and projecting sound. Without a relaxed abdomen and smooth-functioning diaphragm, we will not have the power to expand our voice. Exercises to build your breath capacity, free your diaphragm from tension and breathe to support projecting your voice are described at the end of this chapter.

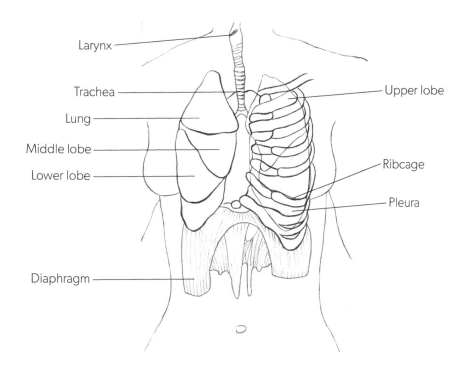

Larynx and vocal folds

Our vocal folds are located within the larynx, sometimes called a vocal tract or, most commonly, voice box. It's not at all shaped like a box, but it might help to think of it as a container. The larynx sits between vertebrae C4 and C6 and is made up of cartilage structures that provide attachment points for the vocal folds. A very simple image to visualize this is to think of the neck and the cartilage structures as the frame of a harp, and the vocal folds inside like the strings of the harp. The larynx's main job is *phonation*, or the creation of sound. It also helps to protect the upper respiratory tract, working as a filter.

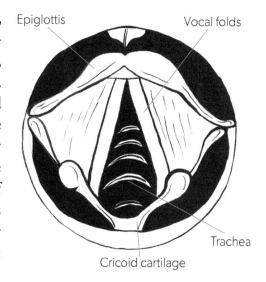

The muscles around the larynx control the length and shape of the vocal folds, which is what makes pitch and tone. Imagine this metaphoric harp has a frame that moves and changes shape. Men, women and children have different sized vocal folds, which is why our larynxes are also different sizes. The larger larynx and vocal folds in an adult male create a typically lower-pitched voice. Size and structure are not the only factors when it comes to the pitch of the voice. How we use the larynx is also extremely important in creating and manipulating pitch, and this is where training and practice can help us to improve our vocal ability and our range of possibilities.

Genetics play a large role in the way we sound, helping to determine not only the size and shape of our vocal tract and vocal folds, but also the ability and speed with which they come together (adduction) or move apart (abduction). Just as we learn to train the body in yoga asana, the breath in prānāyāma and the mind with meditation, it is practice that provides a path to changing our personal attitudes toward our voices and this is the key to improving our ability to project and our sound.

The glottis

This refers to the anatomy above the larynx that is involved in shaping sound into language or music: the tongue, the teeth, the glottis (it looks like a tiny punching bag at the back of the throat when you open your mouth really wide), the gums, the jaw, the cheek, the palates (both hard and soft) and the lips. These work to help the air and vibrations to become sound, as well as literally shaping that sound. When we articulate well, we are using these parts of the body to make our sounds clear. *Articulation* is similar 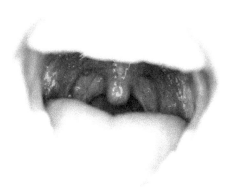 to *enunciation*, but in the world of speech and voice training they are not exactly the same. Articulation is the use of the parts listed above, and enunciation is saying words clearly. We must articulate well in order to enunciate our words.

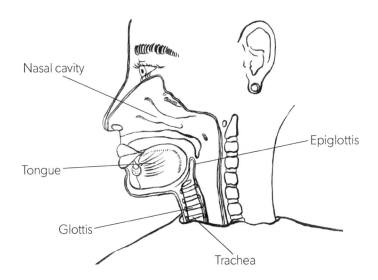

Resonators

These are the parts of your body that influence your ability to project sound. They are the empty or hollow areas that I think of as little caves. When you send your voice through a cave it bounces back at you, and the shape and depth of the cave affect the way your sound comes back: louder, softer, farther away, closer, parts of the word echoing. When we make sound it passes through these open spaces in the body, and as it passes it resonates or becomes amplified so the sound can travel. Resonance can refer to improving sound—making it louder or more esthetically pleasing—or to a feeling of emotional resonance. Words associated with vocal resonance include amplification, enrichment, enlargement, improvement and intensification. Physically, resonance occurs in your body when sound moves through your head, mouth, chest and nose. Clearly, the shape of these body parts influences the sounds you make. These different physical areas are used to create certain moods and tones, as well as volume. As an example, when we focus on resonating through the chest the sound is warmer and might be described as heartfelt; the chest is also a bigger space to create a louder sound.

Many people think the sinuses are only part of the nasal cavity; however, we have four pairs of sinuses: maxillary (cheek), ethmoid (nasal), frontal (forehead) and sphenoid (back of the head). The sinuses have a very interesting structure, with an interior like a honeycomb matrix of soft tissues that produce mucus and react to the air around you. When your sinuses are blocked, you sound completely different from when they are clear.

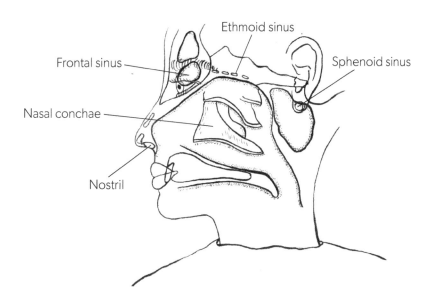

The most effective area for amplifying sound in your body is your pharynx, the space at the back of your throat behind the mouth and nasal cavity and above the larynx and esophagus. This space is totally affected by the state of the muscles around it—think of the harp. The muscles around the pharynx are connected with your cervical spine, as you can see in the diagram. This is why your ability to project your voice is influenced by the tension levels of your neck, shoulders, jaw and facial muscles. In some cases of extreme tension in these areas, even small sounds are impossible.

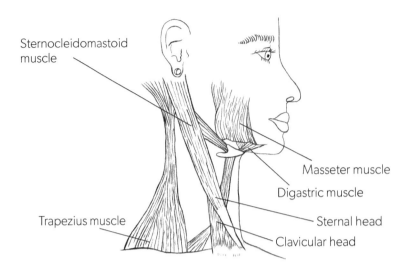

Sternocleidomastoid muscle

Masseter muscle

Digastric muscle

Trapezius muscle

Sternal head

Clavicular head

POSTURE: THE PRIMARY FOUNDATION

You probably have an idea of posture that might have judgments attached like "good" or "bad." I know I do. It's interesting that in the West we focus so much on physical yoga postures, yet many of us are not tuned in to our posture off the mat. Since each person has an individual body and history, posture is something that we must look at through the lens of "neutral" or "optimal function" rather than allowing the dual-focused attitude of "good/bad" to bias the way we work with our own bodies and those of others. Osteopathic clinical researcher Michael Kuchera has a definition of posture that I appreciate:

> Posture is distribution of body mass in relation to gravity over a base of support. The efficiency with which weight is distributed over the base of support depends on the levels of energy needed to maintain equilibrium (homeostasis), as well as on the status of the musculo-ligamentous structures of the body.[3]

EXERCISES AS EXPLORATION: STARTING TO PRACTICE

The status of our musculoligamentous structures is affected by hormones, gravity, strength, age and a variety of other factors. In an ideal world our asana practice helps to improve our posture off the mat, giving us a structure that is more balanced. It is important that you notice the type of practice you have and take into account whether or not your asana practice is improving your musculoskeletal imbalances or increasing them. For the typically flexible, hypermobile or hormonally influenced ligaments (during ovulation, menstruation, pregnancy and lactation women experience higher levels of the hormone relaxin, which increases the laxity of ligaments throughout the body) we must make the choice to find stability in asana rather than exploiting flexibility.

Many traditional yoga practices have an emphasis on stretching the posterior (back) chain of the body, and some do not include abdominal strengthening. As we look at common postural issues, I encourage you to study yourself and create a practice that helps to create ease of movement and better posture throughout the day and hopefully over your lifetime. It is always best to work in person with a teacher and not depend only on self-study. Here are some common postural issues and yoga sequences to help improve them.

Forward head posture (FHP)

This is the most common postural habit. With the head forward of the torso, creating overworked shoulder and neck muscles, a shortened cervical curve develops as well as an exaggerated thoracic curve. This combination makes good vocal projection and sound practically impossible!

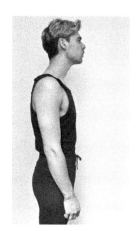

Text neck

This position is common now that smart phones have become so popular. The shortening of the front of the neck puts pressure on the larynx. When the back of the neck is in a lengthened position while bearing weight, as the muscles are asked to hold the head up from gravity, a tension pattern takes over that is also problematic for healthy voice production.

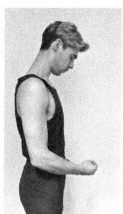

Anterior pelvic tilt

Looking at the line of the waistband on the trousers you can clearly see how the front of the pelvis is tipped downward at an extreme angle. Each unique skeleton has its own "neutral" position. However, when the front of the pelvis tips enough to cause strain along the back and shoulder muscles, we can assume that the pelvis is tilting out of neutral.

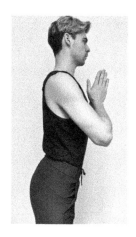
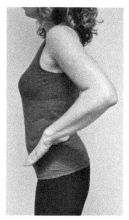

Posterior pelvic tilt

This is less common. However, many yogis have been told that they have too much anterior pelvic tilt and so the habit of "tucking the tail" repeatedly in yoga poses can sometimes become a habit during daily life. If a regular yoga practice includes this tilted position in poses where the spine is meant to be "neutral" (think of tadasana), another tension pattern develops. The front of the abdomen becomes blocked and the pelvic floor is in a position that does not invite proper function. Often the shoulders also round forward with this pelvic position.

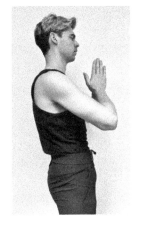
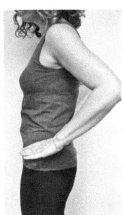

Neutral spine

Remember, we are looking for stability, natural muscle function for upright movement and also a sense of mobility being effortless. Everyone has their own neutral. However, we can look at the spine for guidance on what are normal curves.

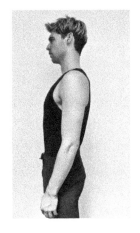
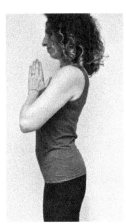

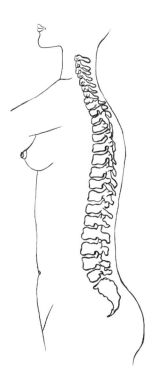

STEPPING ONTO THE PATH

To get comfortable with your voice and this journey, I want you to record yourself reading out the instructions for the exercises. I know for some, the idea of listening to ourselves makes us want to run screaming from the room. Please be gentle with yourself as you take this first step. We all start somewhere. Read the instructions slowly, so that you will have time to do them as you practice. It works really well for most of the exercises to have a timer set up nearby so that you can let go of watching the clock. There's nothing less relaxing or distracting than wondering what time it is!

The following yoga poses are helpful in developing good postural habits and help develop your breath awareness and capacity. We will get into the vocal exercises during the next chapter. Beginning to identify what poses your body needs is part of this first step in looking at yourself with kind eyes and moving in the direction of letting go of your blocks.

Recommended props:

- 1 sticky mat

- 3 blankets

- 2 blocks

- 1 yoga belt.

Constructive rest

This pose is for finding a neutral spinal position when you are horizontal with gravity in order to experience as little tension as possible throughout your body. It is used in many practices, and I love its power to help us release the diaphragm and psoas in particular. It takes some time to learn where your body is most comfortable.

Lie on the floor with a sticky mat for your feet, but as many blankets as you like under the rest of your body. Take care that your head and pelvis are evenly supported by any blankets or padding you use before you place the first head support layer. With a simple blanket fold under your head so that your neck feels comfortable and slightly lengthened, the chin comes to a neutral position, pointing neither up nor down. If your sacrum is tender or you have any lower back discomfort, try a small cushion or another blanket under your pelvis. If your hip flexors are very tight, try a yoga belt around your thighs to rest into. Start with your knees bent and feet about hip width apart, and test your feet slightly closer, slightly farther away, perhaps turning in or out a little. Take some time to try each foot position with a breath before testing another, looking for the most restful position to feel more of the foot on the mat as opposed to only resting on sections. Some people like the feet turned in a bit. For some, internal rotation of the thigh bones at the hip sockets is preferable, while others prefer the opposite. For some, the legs rest better with the feet farther away from the pelvis; for others, it is better with the feet closer. Try a slight change in any of these directions. Take a breath and feel. Your body will tell you what it needs. Listen and trust. Look for a feeling of spreading weight widely and evenly through all areas of your bones rather than sinking down on one part. Create a sense of ease in the joints by placing your arms wide enough that there is space around the upper ribs and armpits. Make sure you are warm enough to stay here for about 15 minutes. This pose uses gravity to release muscular tension and help our bones align well, which takes time. Maybe you need some music for this time, or a podcast that is inspiring or a guided meditation. Maybe you can rest in silence and use this pose to meditate. See what works for you and know that staying longer is the only way to find true results.

HELPFUL YOGA POSES FOR FHP

Constructive rest with belly breathing and knees together modification

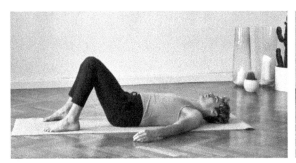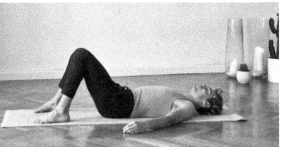

Notice the subtle change of the abdomen on inhale and exhale. Instead of using muscular effort to keep the pelvis still, the pelvis will move freely with the breath and affect the entire spine in a subtle rocking when you are deeply relaxed here.

Chest opening variation with cactus arms

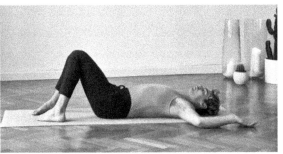

If the area around your thoracic spine is very tight, you might want a layer of extra padding under your head. You might notice this tension if your chin points up and the cervical curve is shortened. It is very likely if you have FHP when standing that you would have this tension pattern when lying supine.

Feet elevated variation

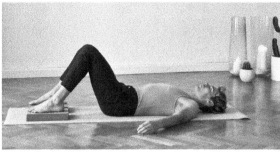

Try different levels and textures for your feet to find what helps your lumbar curve move toward neutral. If you have a strong anterior tilt, this might work well to help the pelvis shift.

Bolster on the toes

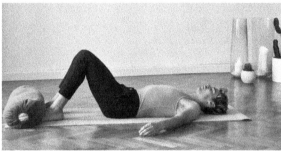

My personal favorite. This variation gives a lot of grounding and helps the feet to relax.

Feet on the bolster

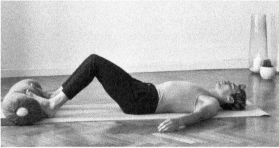

This is a great option to help very tight hip flexors release. Another one to try if you tend to have a strong anterior pelvic tilt.

Strap around the thighs

 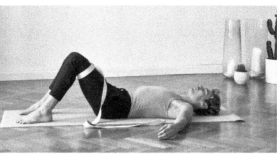 

This is great for any S-I (sacro-iliac joint) or pelvic instability. It also helps the hip flexor area and can be easier to relax into than the previous option.

Make it restorative

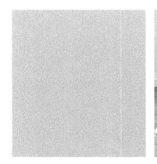 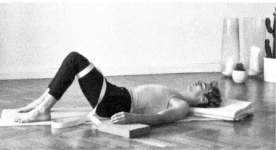 

Adding blocks or books under the wrist and hand helps release shoulder tension. This is my favorite position for the arm in relaxation poses. Your elbow is on the floor and the shoulder joint is in a neutral rotational position.

The blanket is placed with the corner under C7 (see the photo at the bottom of page 38), allowing the neck optimal length without stretching. This is very effective in helping all postural habits improve. To complete this as a full restorative pose, add an eye cover for darkness and a blanket for warmth.

Passive bridge with block

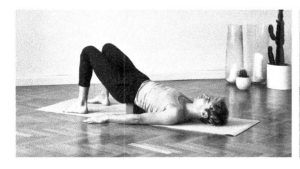 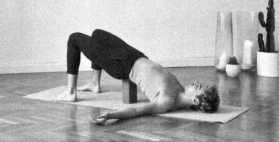

Place the block under your sacrum at a height that allows your back to relax. This position is fantastic for increasing your abdominal space and ability to belly breathe. When using the block on the taller setting, make sure the block is not only on the sacrum but also supporting the ilium. This prevents overstretching of the ligaments at the S-I joints.

Hip flexor release with core stability

Explore extending one leg while keeping the sacrum and shoulders centered rather than allowing gravity to pull you to one side. The heel on the extended leg remains on the floor and the foot active so the leg is neutral in rotation at your hip socket. Try cactus arms. If you need a deeper stretch, draw the opposite knee in, and keep the sacrum and shoulders even.

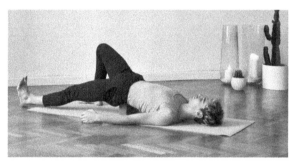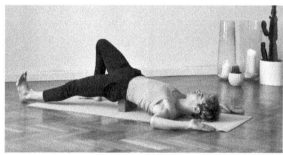
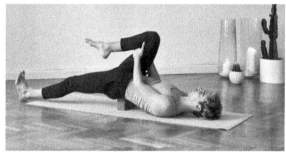

Bridge pose: traditional arm position

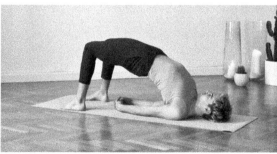

Bridge pose: robot arms variation

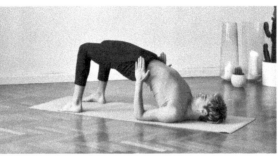

This is effective to help build strength and awareness in the latissimus dorsi muscles as well as helping to feel the power of using the upper body to keep the weight from collapsing into the lower back. I find this version allows me to feel more specificity in the thoracic spine.

Bridge pose: passive arms variation

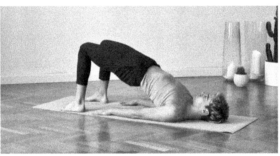

More than a preparation for the other arm variations, this version is helpful in strengthening the legs and posterior chain.

Simple twist with open legs

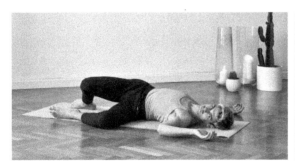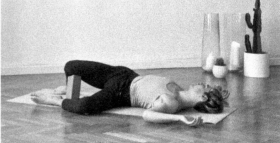

This is a variation of the simple supine twist where you leave your feet at the edges of the yoga mat. Try it with either cactus arms or extended arms. If you experience any knee sensitivity, use the block as shown in the second photo. The block is also useful if you are staying in the pose longer to help release hip flexor and groin tension.

As a flowing option, go slowly to get a massage along the back of your pelvis from the pressure of the ground. Work on releasing into the ground and moving in rhythm with your breath. The same goes for the movement of the head, which can be in opposition to or the same direction as the legs. Use the eyes to follow a line that keeps the neck long and the chin neutral. Do both sides evenly unless you find one side of your body is tighter, in which case give it more time to release and stretch!

Downward dog with forehead or crown of head on block

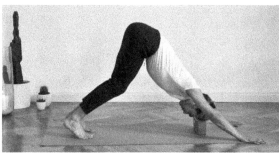

For this to release the neck muscles you need to clearly feel you are resting your head on the support, as opposed to feeling the block is pressing your head closer to your body. Try different block variations (or books) to get the height exactly right for you.

Dolphin (forearm dog pose)

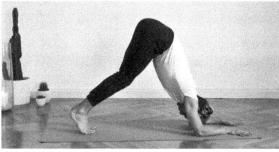

The most important thing here is to keep the elbows directly under your shoulders so you can lift from between the shoulder blades and make space for your head to hang down without touching the ground. The idea is for gravity to traction your neck and let it hang.

Prasarita padotanasana variation

This variation uses a strap to help focus on stretching the front of the shoulders and opening the chest.

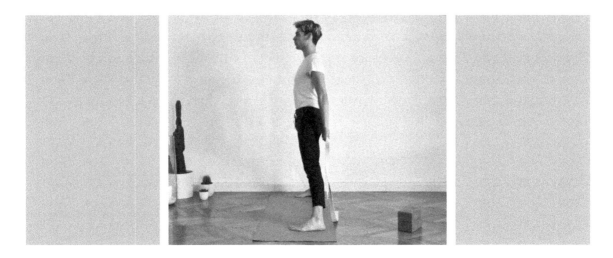

Pay close attention to keeping the hips aligned with the ankles and allowing the pelvis to rotate smoothly over the heads of the femurs.

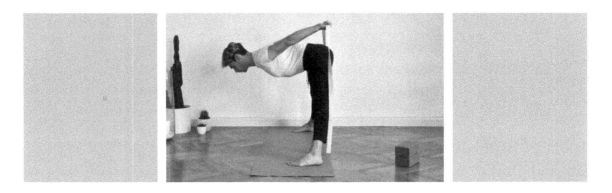

You might feel this as more of a leg stretch, so check that you are not pushing too far toward the head and losing the effect on the shoulders. If your legs are too tight to find the shoulder stretch, try bending the knees.

   When the shoulders are open enough to clasp your hands together and keep the elbows straight then you might try this variation without the strap. The strap offers more access to opening the shoulders, try both when you are ready.

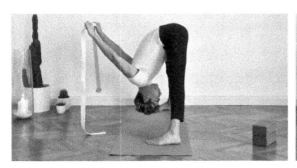
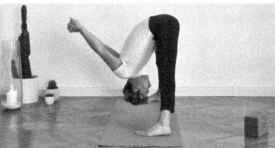

Inversions

Take care when practicing inversions to make sure your body is prepared. This means you need to have a level of shoulder and thoracic spine mobility, as well as the strength and coordination to do the pose safely. The following inversions will be held with the spine in neutral, which means that to counter gravity you have to work the pelvis so that the frontal hip points (I will refer to the anterior superior iliac spine (ASIS) as hip points throughout the book) move toward the low ribs. Your neck should remain long and your breath remain steady. Avoid these poses if you have a neck or spinal injury, or are pregnant or menstruating.

Headstand

Take the time to set your foundation well for this pose. Follow each step to help core awareness. Keeping the neck extended and looking for length along the spine is the aim. To be safe 70 percent of your weight is in your hands/forearms and the head never bears more than 30 percent. Feel free to start at the wall if this is not a familiar pose for you. Feel free to do a tripod variation directly from your prasarita padotanasana.

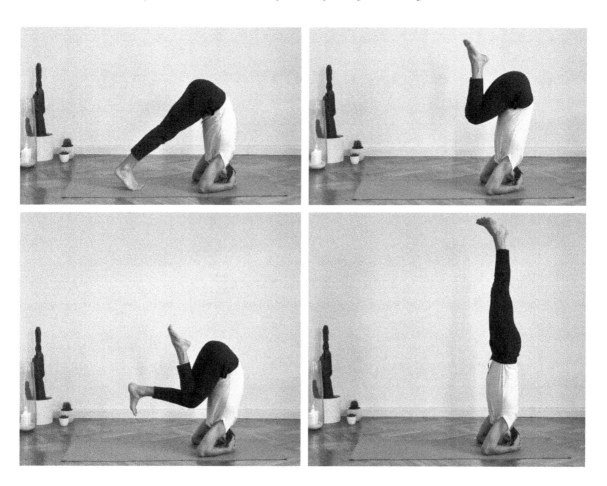

Tripod variation of headstand

Check that you enter and exit with care.

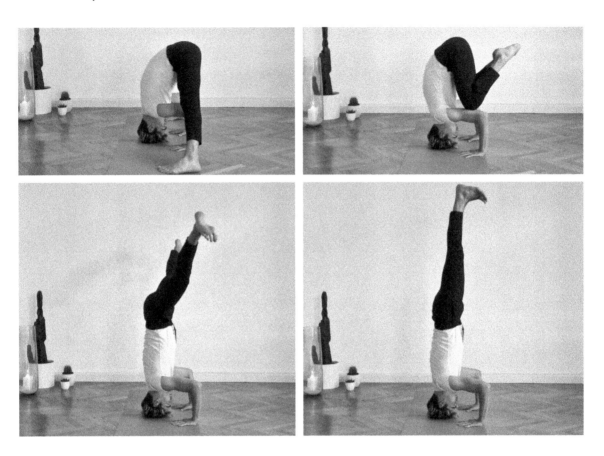

Shoulder stand

Setting up your shoulder stand props can be an exercise in mindfulness. Remember that the props serve an important purpose here: protecting your neck! Too much pressure on the neck in the pose can be very destabilizing for the ligaments at the back of your neck. Take care that the neck has its natural curve in this pose as opposed to a flattened position!

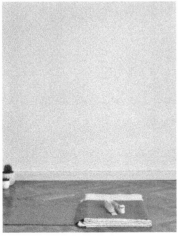 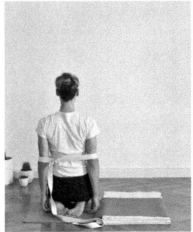 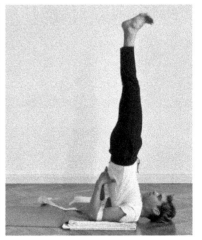

Plow

Aim to feel again the work of the thoracic spine and with your hands lift the pelvis up toward the ceiling. If we focus too much on bringing the feet down, we will risk the spine going into deep flexion, and extension is the aim.

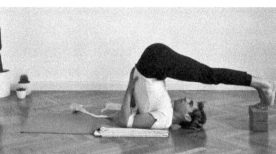

Paschimotanasana with head on block

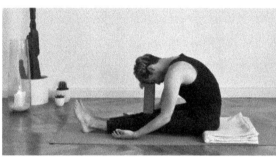

Keep the heels of the feet pressing forward to engage the legs with a parallel hip rotation. Be mindful that the legs do not work so hard that the heels come off the floor.

Janu sirsasana with head on block

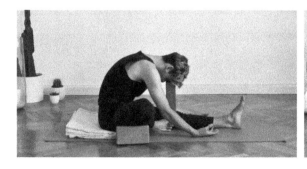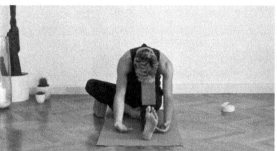

This can be done with as many props as you need to create relaxation along the back of the body.

This version should give you a lengthening stretch for the back of the leg while relaxing as opposed to stretching the back and neck.

Savasana

I am passionate about savasana, and my work in restorative yoga has shown me that using more props and leaving 15–20 minutes for my savasana has taught me to relax on and off the mat. Below is a detailed photo tutorial of how to support the head, neck and shoulders in savasana or many supine restorative postures. Please take time to teach yourself how to do this well. Of course, having a teacher or helper to tuck the blanket in for you is lovely. However, learning to create comfort for ourselves is also vital. Enjoy!

All blankets have a different personality; cotton blankets that don't slip are easiest. This is the fold you start with.

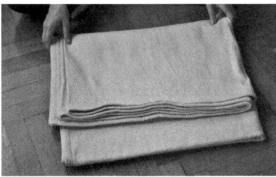

Making sure that the bottom layer of the blanket only supports the top of the upper trapezius (not the whole scapula), it should end at the "spine of the scapula." Vertebra C7 should rest on the top section of blanket edges.

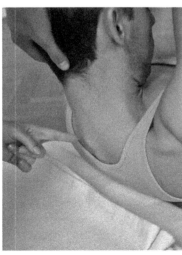
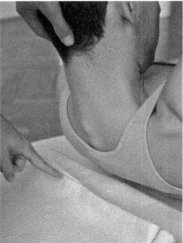

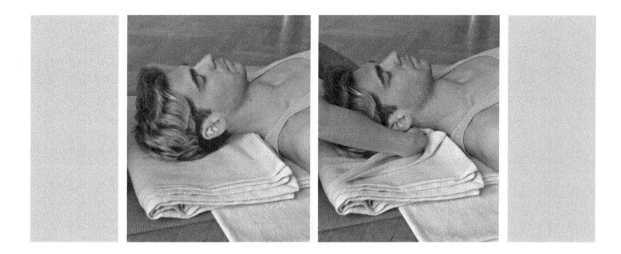

Starting with the top layer, take each blanket layer and fold it under as you firmly stuff it along your neck and shoulders. Be careful *not* to lift or move your head as you tuck yourself in. The blanket should mold to your body like papier mâché. The more time you take to separate each layer before stuffing in the blanket, the firmer it will be and the better it will feel!

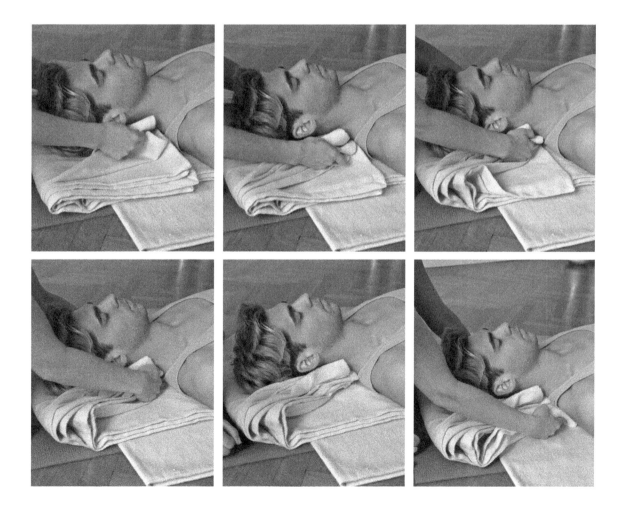

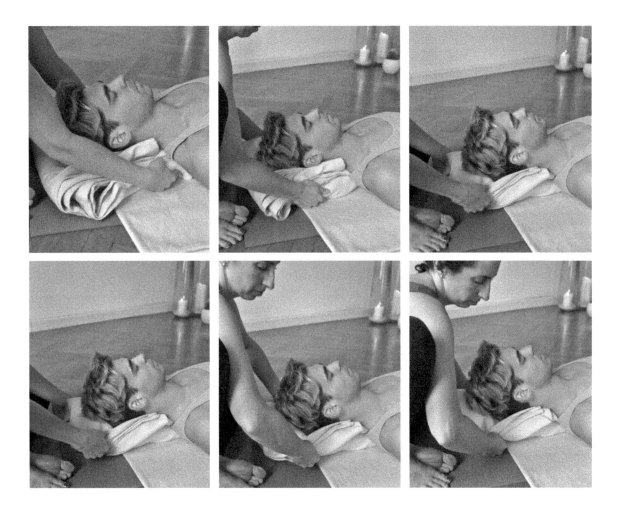

When the blanket is tucked all around the head, the top of the blanket folds under with enough height to lift the back of the skull so that it tilts at an angle. This *slightly* stretches the back of the neck so there is no sensation of stretch, only relaxation. If the chin points up toward the ceiling, perhaps add a thin layer of extra blanket or a book or yoga brick under the back of the skull to achieve the optimal position for the head.

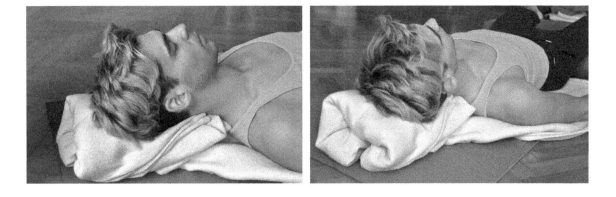

This blanket folding also has the effect of creating a release for the shoulders and an openness in the chest.

 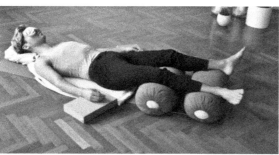 

Full savasana with props for deep relaxation

 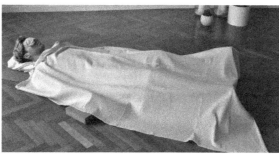 

Cover yourself with a blanket to stay warm and rest for 15–20 minutes, or longer if possible. Use the timer to give yourself permission to truly let go.

GOING INWARD: REFLECTIONS ON FHP SEQUENCE

Take notes on how this practice goes for you. Perhaps you would like to add some poses that help you feel the head centered above the spine. Be honest about how much time you devote to this work. The practices need a gradual increase of time and to be held for a long time to make a noticeable difference.

_____

_____

_____

_____

_____

_____

_____

_____

_____

CORE WORK TO IMPROVE STRENGTH FOR SPINAL STABILITY

This is a mini sequence to use within any other sequence you choose. It is also good to do on its own if you are short of time.

Dolphin plank

Aim to hold this for 20 slow breaths. Keep the lumbar curve extended by actively tucking your tail under and bringing all of the work to the abdominal muscles rather than the back muscles.

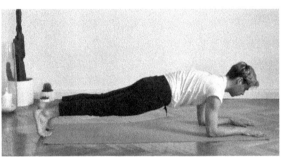

Plank

Again, focus on the lower back staying flat, and by lifting slightly between the shoulder blades you bring more focus to the abdominals.

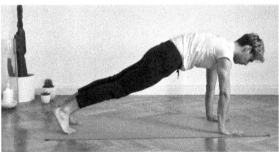

Side plank

Stay on the edges of the feet with both feet fully flexed. Draw the bottom shoulder away from the ear. Watch that the top hip stays level with the bottom hip.

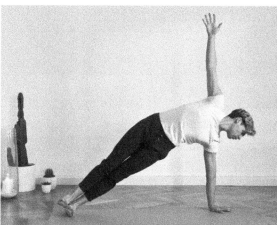

Side plank variation

Try this version if you cannot hold the body straight in the previous version. Keep the knee 90°, lined up with the hip and ankle.

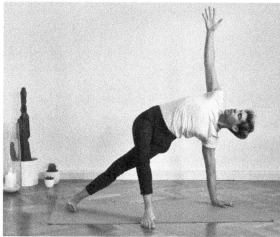

Inversions are a fantastic way to strengthen the core! Adding the inversions (headstand, tripod headstand, shoulder stand) as described earlier in this chapter and practiced with good alignment requires and builds core awareness in any sequence.

SEQUENCE TO HELP RELEASE ANTERIOR PELVIC TILT

Another mini sequence that can be combined with other practices or perhaps choosing one of these poses to focus on will help you move in the direction of a neutral pelvis. I like to start with sun salutations to warm up for these poses. Refer to the section headed "Hip flexor release with core stability" at the bottom of page 31.

Lunges at the wall

These intense stretches for the hip flexors will also work on your quadriceps and psoas. Take care to pad the back knee properly and avoid this if your knees are injured or sensitive. If it is not possible for your knees, modify by moving away from the wall (see below) and keeping the back leg engaged so that you are not allowing gravity to pull you down. The work is to keep the frontal hip points reaching up toward the lower ribs, so that you are actively moving out of an anterior tilt of the pelvis! Please be gentle with these and take care to stay with an intensity level that allows for deep steady breath. Notice how the shoulders are moving away from the ears, the collar bones are widening and the neck is long.

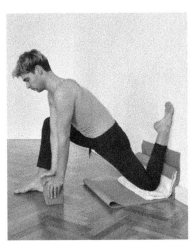
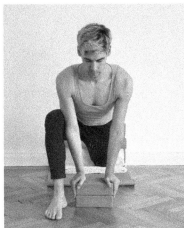
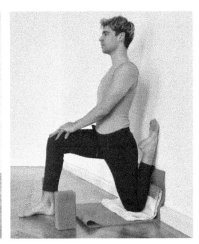

Lunges off the wall

Taking care again with the hip points, use the same alignment principles as when you work at the wall. Avoid dropping the frontal hip area by giving in to gravity, even when this means making the pose smaller and backing off!

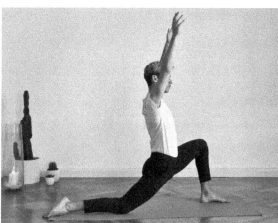

King Arthur

I'm not sure why this pose has this name; however, it is the most effective stretch I know for stretching tight hip flexors, a major cause of anterior pelvic tilt.

The pelvis does not need to come all the way to the wall. As you move from the previous lunges toward bringing your pelvis to the wall you will find the appropriate places to pause along the way and breathe. When you are able to bring your pelvis to the wall (it might take a lifetime), watch that it remains neutral in the coronal plane (anatomy speak for keeping the right and left sides of the pelvis level). Notice the "no no" photo of scrunching up the shoulders. No shoulder tension! When the shoulders scrunch we often let the low ribs flare open. Keep the low ribs and frontal hip points reaching together to have neutral spinal curves.

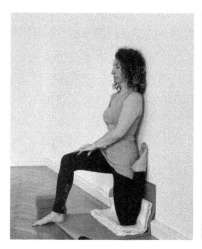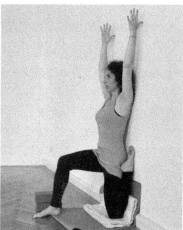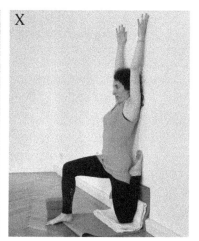

Ustrasana at the wall: step by step

Notice how important it is in this version to keep the hip points against the wall as a full step or even the entire pose. This requires a lot of core strength and moving slowly in and out of the pose. Watch the length of your neck, favor a feeling of working with the whole spine and avoid sensations of specific tension in the lower back. Aim for giving yourself a few times with this pose, resting with the face in each direction after.

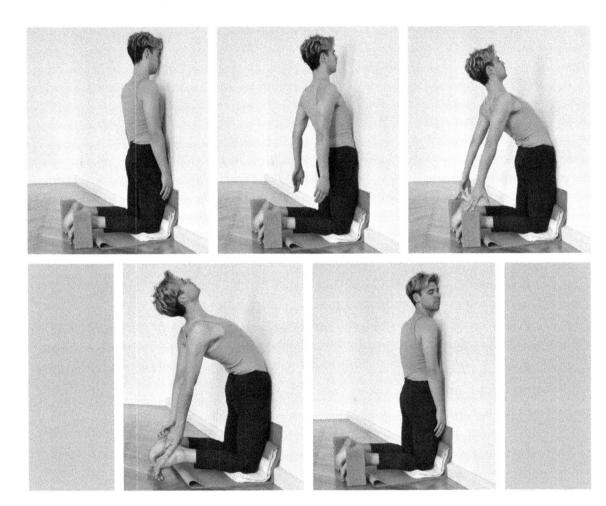

Virbhadrasana II

This is a great test for the pelvic tilt, if you pay attention to the front hip staying level with the back hip (neutral in the coronal plane). A fun trick is to wedge your fingers into the front hip crease. If you can't get in there, chances are you are tilting too much of your pelvis toward your front leg. Work more on the front hip lifting up.

 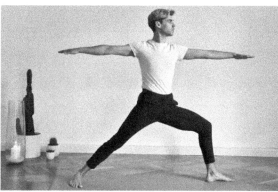 

Urdhva dhanurasana from constructive rest

Make sure to follow the proper slow entry technique in these photos. Try three rounds and explore staying longer in the pose while breathing smoothly. Coming down, reverse the entry technique and take time to stay in constructive rest with your spine neutral before any other pose. Follow with twists before forward folding. Cool down poses are necessary after such a large shape. Try the open twists before adding the forward folds in the previous sequence.

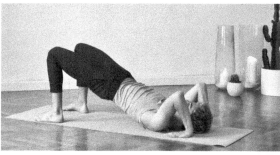 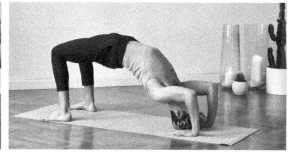

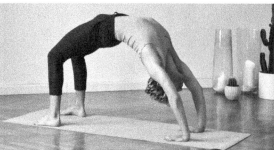 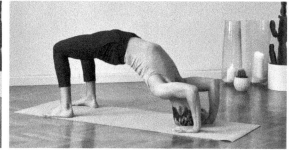

Urdhva dhanurasana on bolsters

The passive version of this pose can be a lovely way to release the psoas. It also works well on a large Pilates ball. Take care with your neck. Stay ten breaths if possible, building up your stamina slowly. Experiment with being passive only when your lower back agrees. If the lower back is not comfortable, modify with bending the knees and keep the feet engaged on the floor. To enter the pose begin with bent knees, lift the pelvis and tuck the tail actively, then lower slowly one vertebra at a time so you come into the pose with a longer lumbar spine. Relax into the bolsters to stay. Bend the knees again and exit by reversing the way you entered, supporting the head with your hands to keep the neck safe.

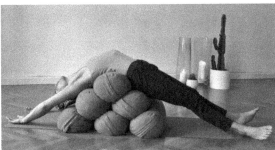

Pigeon on props

By using a prop under the front hip you can once more draw the frontal hips up toward the lower ribs. This requires a lot of internal engagement and will perhaps change the areas that you feel most in this pose. Feel free to try any combination of props, bolsters, blankets and/or blocks. Bolsters are my favorite.

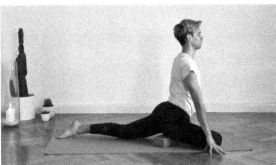

Savasana or constructive rest variations

Choose which pose gives the most open feeling through your lower belly and hips. Here are a couple of reminders that I love. Look back through the chapter for more options.

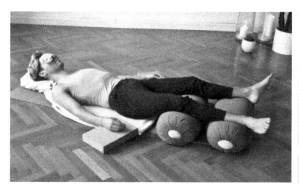 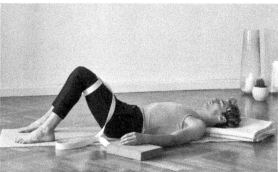

SEQUENCE TO HELP RELEASE POSTERIOR PELVIC TILT

Focus on poses that help you rediscover your lumbar curve and neutral pelvic tilt by releasing buttocks and abdomen. This is often the opposite of what you might have trained your body to do, especially if you were told in the past that your spine was overly lordotic, your ballet teacher told you your behind was large or maybe you are self-conscious of your belly and learned to suck it in.

Constructive rest

Use any variation from the menu of options and photos to find the optimal rest and reset position that encourages lumbar curve during relaxation.

 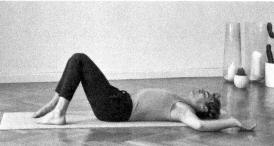 

Restorative backbend: elevated legs prānāyāma savasana

Fold a blanket in thirds, like an accordion. Place the uneven side toward the bolsters for your lumbar curve to be supported.

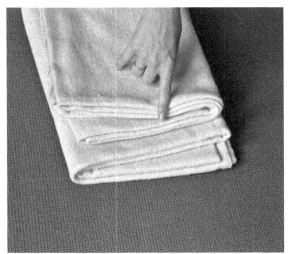 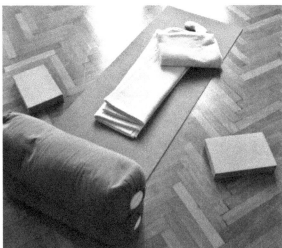

This is a fantastic pose for encouraging the belly to release (hence it is called prānāyāma savasana), and combined with elevating legs with the angle of hip to knee about 45°, it creates a further release in the lower back.

 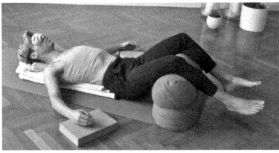 

Follow the instructions for savasana hand support and blanket folding and tucking for the head, neck and shoulders described earlier in this chapter. Cover yourself with a blanket for warmth to stay and enjoy, ideally for 20 minutes.

Restorative backbend with elevated legs and strap on legs

The blanket(s) should start at the bottom ribs and end at the edge of the pelvis. The lumbar spine should feel supported, not shortened. Lift the pelvis and tuck the tail, then slowly release in. Use thinner or fewer blankets if needed. Try this before moving on to three blanket backbend.

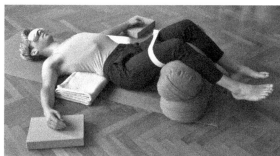

Bolster-free option

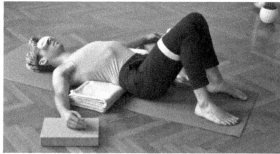

Three blanket backbend

As with the previous backbend, your landmarks for the blankets are the lower ribs and the top rim of the pelvis. Your shoulder blades might touch the blanket, but only at the bottom tip of the scapula. Check your scapulae are off the blankets to release the shoulders and chest.

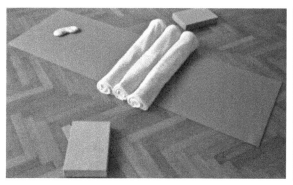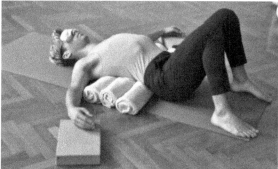

Urdhva dhanurasana on bolsters

 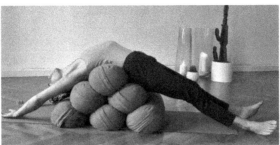 

Bridge with block under sacrum

 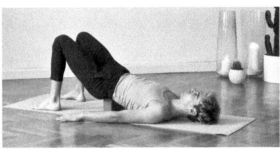 

To end the sequence, repeat prānāyāma savasana or any savasana you enjoy.

POSES TO DISCOVER AND STRENGTHEN NEUTRAL CURVES

Tadasana

Playing with balance, try rocking your weight slightly forward, sideways and then back in order to find a true center. Work with a mirror, a teacher or a friend. Try it also with your eyes closed to feel how the abdomen stabilizes your spine in relation to your feet. Try tadasana lying down with active arms and legs, noticing your spinal curves.

 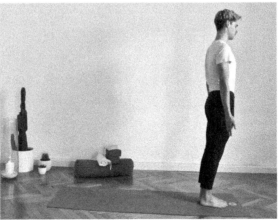 

Uttitha hastasana

As you raise your arms, notice if you tend toward a posterior or anterior pelvic tilt. Stabilize to remain more neutral. It's helpful to have a mirror partner for honest feedback. Keep in mind that each body has its own neutral.

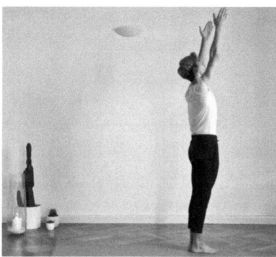

Uttkatasana

Focus again on keeping neutrality in the spine. Avoid the temptation of tucking under or flaring the ribs. Move slowly so you can feel where your spine is familiar with bearing the stress of gravity and you can shift the stress to create a more head to toe physical effort.

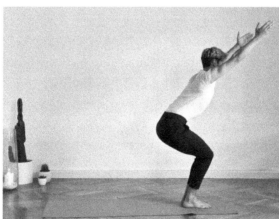

Prāṇāyāma

I recommend you continue your prāṇāyāma practice in constructive rest (see pages 27–30), or a semi-reclined restorative pose where your back is fully supported when you begin. As your prāṇāyāma practice develops you can use seated poses where you are able to remain upright with comfort. Traditionally, breathing practices are done after the asana practice, with a break in-between. All of these breath practices need to be done with a quality of softness and ease in the body, which will help you to focus and gives the mind the quality of ease as well. This is how prāṇāyāma helps to shift our nervous system toward the parasympathetic. The practices of Bhrāmerī and Kapālabhātī wake up the nervous system, so if you are anxious do not use them as they might not help you to feel calmer. Some people find breath retention or any focus on breathing can lead to sensations of anxiety. If this happens for you please release any controlling technique and stay with breath awareness or simply take a break. Respect the message that your body sends and do not use force.

T.K.V. Desikachar writes in his book *The Heart of Yoga*:

> The most important tenet of prananyama is this: Only when we have emptied ourselves can we take in a new breath, and only when we can draw the breath into us can we hold it. If we cannot breathe out and in fully, how are we going to hold our breath? Breath-retention exercises must be done in such a way that they never disturb the in- and out-breaths. When we reach the stage where we have improved our ability to breathe in and out and to hold the breath, then breath-retention may become important because as it is held the breath is at rest, and with it so hopefully is the mind.[4]

Breath awareness

To focus on the movement of the diaphragm, touch your belly as you breathe. Touch your skin so you have a more tactile experience of the body breathing. Pay attention to releasing tension from the abdomen and tuning in to the feelings of pressure changing along your pelvic floor with the inhale and exhale. Ideally after some time you will remember how to breathe in a relaxed and deep way.

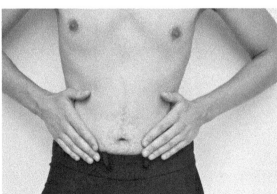

Lateral breath awareness

Bring your hands to the side ribs (along the seam where a T-shirt would be sewn together). Feel the way your body opens like an accordion with the inhale and settles back in with the exhale. Imagine the inter-costal muscles (the muscles between the ribs) gently stretching open on inhale, the bottom of the lungs blossoming outwards. Tune in and be curious about where you feel your body moves and has space.

Do keep your face relaxed.

Don't try to breathe faster or harder, which tenses the face and lips.

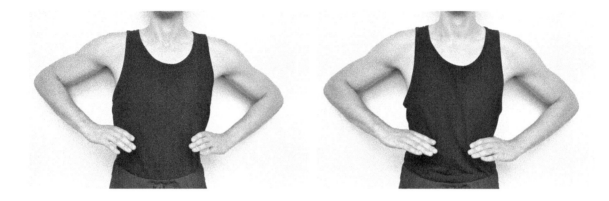

Straw breathing

You can practice breathing (slowly) through a straw as a tool for helping you track your lung capacity, rhythm and sensations during breath. This is a very effective way of sidetracking the mind and getting to a truly diaphragmatic breath. This can be very helpful for asthma, chest breathing and those of us who are not used to completing the exhale.

Try a few rounds of four breaths to get used to the feeling.

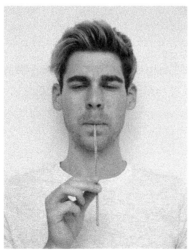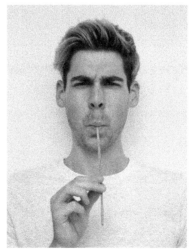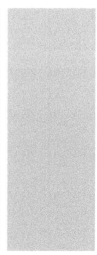

Śītalī/sītkārī: cooling breath

Breathing along the tongue on the inhale cools the breath, then breathing out through the nose helps the body release heat. Some of us can easily curl the tongue to create a narrow, straw-like passage for the breath to come into the body. Take care to purse the lips gently, without over-tensing the face! For genetic reasons some of us cannot curl the tongue and will simply rest the tip of the tongue gently on the back of the bottom teeth. This method has an equally cooling effect.

Inhale the breath through the teeth along the tongue as you gently lift your chin. Stay within your end range of movement, keeping the back of the neck easy. Exhale from the nose and lower your chin back to neutral. With your breath slow and steady, aim for 8 to 12 rounds.

Viloma I: focusing breath

This helps to build breath capacity and familiarize our ribcage with bigger movement during breath. It also increases our ability to breathe low, toward the belly, which is ideal for keeping the diaphragm free and our breath effortless during speech. This is thought to help depressive and lethargic energy shift toward motivation and clarity.

- Exhale fully.

- Inhale only a third of your breath capacity—pause.

- Inhale another third of your breath capacity—pause.

- Inhale the last third of your breath capacity—pause.

Just as in the viloma II practice, keep your face, jaw, throat and shoulders relaxed throughout. The amount of time that you pause is something to work toward building in length.

Viloma II: pacifying breath

By interrupting the exhale, we strengthen our lungs, access the parasympathetic nervous system and practice softening the throat and jaw. This is great for anxiety and also to help focus our thoughts.

- Inhale fully.

- Exhale—pause.

- Exhale—pause.

- Exhale—pause.

As you start you will want a short pause, one that is sustainable while remaining soft through the face/neck/jaw area. When the teeth clench or your body tenses this is the opposite of the effect we are looking for. Increase the time of your pause only as your body is able to remain relaxed and you can keep the shoulders easy throughout the inhale that begins each round. Ten rounds is a lovely place to get to. Begin with whatever you can manage and build up slowly. When you finish please take some time to notice the effect.

Kapālabhātī: shining skull or pumping breath

This is helpful for cleansing the mucus or any blockages from the airways and sinuses. It can also release tension from the chest and throat. It is called shining skull breath as it is meant to shift energy up toward the top of the head.

Take a full breath in to begin, with one hand on your lower belly (above the pubic bone, below the navel). With sharp, strong, short exhales begin to contract the lower belly toward the spine. This pumps the air out of your lungs with short exhales. Let the inhales come passively as a response to the vacuum created from the short exhales. Give yourself around eight to ten sharp exhales and then a slow deep inhale before starting the next round.

Bhrāmerī: the humming bumble bee breath

One of my favorites as it helps clear the sinuses and energize the body. A fantastic warm-up for the vocal cords and jaw.

Inhale smoothly to fill the lungs completely. Exhale with relaxed jaw and lips lightly touching as you create a humming sound. Move the sound from the tingling of the lips around the head, and down the throat and into the chest. Change the pitch of your voice to change the place you feel the vibration. Play with where you get the most power from the hum, starting softly and getting as loud as you want to help build confidence in making sound.

Nadi shodhana: alternate nostril breathing

I like this as a mind balancing breath—very helpful for anxiety and low energy. You can physically block off the nostrils using the fingers but be sure to keep the pressure light and not forceful. I also enjoy this and often teach it with visualization rather than physical blocking of the nostrils. For the passive version try it lying down in savasana or constructive rest. For depression it is recommended to use the right nostril only, and for anxiety the left. See for yourself what gives you the best result.

Nadi shodhana: traditional hands

Place the thumb above your right nostril and curl your index and middle fingers in toward your palm, resting your ring finger above your left nostril. Inhale and exhale fully to begin through both nostrils. Gently block the right nostril as you inhale from the left, then close the left so both nostrils are closed as you pause briefly. Open the left to exhale and then inhale left to start the next round. Repeat, building up to about ten rounds.

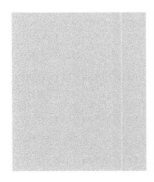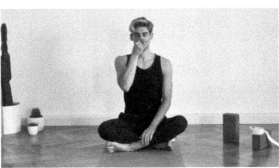

Nadi shodhana: passive arms

I like this version lying down. However, it can also be done sitting. The hands represent what the nostrils are doing, so you do not need to touch your face. It helps build sensory awareness and reminds us that at all times one nostril is most likely dominant!

Take a full breath through both nostrils to begin. Gently close the right hand into a light fist, focusing on the left nostril as you inhale, perhaps even the whole left side of your body. Close the left hand into a light fist and hold the breath in with both fists gently closed. Open the right hand and focus on the right nostril and right side of your body as you exhale. Inhale and keep focusing on the right side and then pause with both hands closed. Exhale out the left as the left hand opens. Repeat, building up to about ten rounds.

MANTRA CHANTING FOR VOCAL HEALTH AND POWER

> In the structure of the creative power of sound, Nada, as Saraswati, is the primordial sound vibration emanating from the kundalini at the base of the spine, parallelling the creation of the universe. She manifests as Pashyanti, or intuitive speech, when emanating from the Swadishthana (second) chakra. As Para, or unmanifested speech, Saraswati springs from the Anahata chakra at the heart center, and extends through the brow center. Thus, her power as sound is contained within us at every level of our being and spiritual development.[5]

Chanting is a beautiful way to connect with making sound. Mantras in Sanskrit have energetic effects beyond simply making sound. The chakra for the throat area has a correlating sound, called the bija, or seed mantra. One way to begin a chanting practice for vocal power is with this mantra.

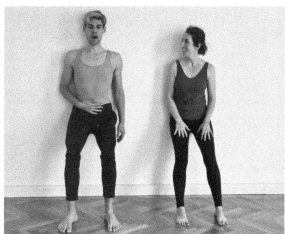

HAM/throat chakra

You can start soft and slow, then gradually build some volume and length as you sing the word HAM. Feel how the throat contracts with the H sound, then opens with the A sound. When you come to the M sound allow the sound to travel back into your body, as if you are swallowing it gently. Notice how the vibration moves back into the body, with a similar feeling to bhrāmerī, a buzzing vibration.

Pro tip

So ham is Sanksrit for "I am." This is a great mantra to chant in the shower with some steam to help the vocal cords before a long day of teaching. Focus on the vibrations as well as getting the mouth to open really big so you stretch your face during this warm-up.

2

WHAT IS VOICE WORK?

The holy grail of voice training is still that unmistakable thrill when the actor speaks and the listener shudders internally with recognition and empathy. Truthfulness and a sense of limitlessness are the goals. The alchemy of inspired communication is a mix of emotion, intellect and voice. The "prima materia" is the breath.

Kristin Linklater

Scientifically, you cannot measure whether a voice has *resonance*, in the figurative meaning of the word. However, as humans we most certainly feel when it does. When a voice resonates with you, the message of the speaker has a stronger effect. In fact, when the voice doesn't resonate, the information might not be absorbed or communicated at all. The definition of *resonate* is both the physical action of resonating and the ability of an idea to be deeply understood. When we want our teaching to resonate with our students, we must also be aware of our physical resonators and whether we are using them to our full advantage. As you learned in the last chapter, how we make sound is a technical process and the more we know and understand the mechanisms of our sound making capabilities, the more we can improve those sounds. The voice work I will explain in this chapter is typically used in theater training for actors. It is different from speech training, which I will get into in the next chapter. I am not a singer and although singing will definitely improve your vocal power, it is a different technique from what you need for speaking. In the accompanying exercises for voice technique that are distinct from yoga and prāṇāyāma, please bear in mind that they are also meant to increase your creative response to impulse and instinct, just as they do for actors. There is much emphasis on breath and freedom, so if you haven't worked in this way before, remember to be extra gentle and compassionate with yourself. In this chapter we will look at the techniques I have used in my theater work and have found effective in helping yoga teachers.

As I continue to research and test different techniques and exercises it has become clear to me that the lineage of voice work and teaching, as I have learned it, is very Anglo-centric. The history of my training is linked to English theater trends. The most common voice work in the English-speaking theater world today can be traced back to Cicely Berry, who was trained at the Central School of Speech and Drama in the voice lineage of the time. Kristin Linklater's teacher at LAMDA, Iris Warren developed a direction of voice work that deviated from that of the Central School and moved the emphasis of the work from that of training a musical instrument to training the whole human by working from outside in to inside out. Much like popular yoga can be traced back to a few main teachers in the last century that brought it to the West, most voice teachers can trace their lineages. As I become more exposed to different languages in performance, I have discovered that there are many other techniques and teaching lineages for different languages. English is a very open-mouthed language, with most of the sounds taking place in the middle or front of the mouth. German, for example, has more sounds coming from the back of the throat and fewer words that stress vowels. It is important to note that my writing and experience is based on the English language, and that if you are working with another language I recommend you pay attention to the different sounds from English phonetics and adapt the exercises to help you become clearer with the sounds of your language. Equally important to think about is your first language, or as my teacher at LISPA used to say often, the "mother tongue." When we work toward freedom of expression, when we peel back the blocks that stand in our way, we want to have the clearest path possible. Practicing some of these exercises in your mother tongue will be a huge help in your creative and expressive process. Even if English is your primary teaching language, give yourself sufficient time to work in your first language and free the mind of the extra step of translation, so that you can access your emotions more easily.

STARTING YOUR VOCAL PRACTICE

One main difference between vocal practice and yoga practice is the intention and use of gravity. In most yoga postures we are engaging against the force of gravity to build strength or increase a stretching of muscle tissue. The aim with our practice for voice work is to find a release of tension. This will take you some time to feel as it is a different sensation from any other. The following exercises are best done with a sense of play. Remember this and, most importantly, to rest when you feel tired. Avoid vocal strain at all times. Your learning process is best done by coming back fresh to try again when you are ready. It doesn't pay to push through discomfort or overwork. This is something I have learned the hard way, and sometimes still need reminding of. I think our culture promotes overwork and places a value on exhaustion. If you bring these beliefs to your voice work you will not get results, you will get pain and perhaps worsen your current habitual way of using your voice. There is no gain from pain when it comes to working on your voice. Please underline this, highlight it, whatever you need to do! Muscle memory is created relatively quickly and most voice work begins with undoing old habits. It is identifying and bringing awareness to tension in order to let it go, finding ways to release the body and open toward the creativity and impulses that come from our inner world that characterizes voice work. As with yoga, we are looking to listen to ourselves in a way that creates an honest relationship with our reality, to see and feel, rather than to push or force. So please, work carefully and slowly to clearly make the new muscle memories you want. Create the patterns that serve you. Here is your mantra for voice work and speaking:

Always with a relaxed and open throat.

Freedom

At this point in time the voice techniques for acting and speaking all have one commonality. They work in different ways toward the same goal. That goal is freedom. As yogis we work with the same concept, the idea of moksha which has been translated from the Sanskrit as freedom or liberation. The yoga philosophy of attaining freedom from the limiting perspective of the ego can be directly linked with the idea of physical and emotional freedom that we work toward in voice training. Artistically, acting has gone through many different styles and at different points in history actors were not expected to sound "natural." Today, however, much value is placed on an actor's believability or truthfulness. Vocal techniques of the past may have focused on supporting more stylized speech, but today's training principles are helpful for teachers or public speakers of all kinds because they help support a natural way of speaking.

I think of freedom as our ability to get out of our own way, which is exactly the state that is needed for any creative endeavor. This state is often described as being in a flow state or a state of ease. When we are not self-conscious, we have the ability to surpass our hang-ups and step into a more powerful and intuitive way of being. The following ideas are all different routes to find that way of being and the physical support for vocal expression. Key in this is understanding the difference between relaxed and released. Often students in my workshops talk about relaxing the muscles of the jaw and neck, and this is important during warm-ups but we need an element of tension to be able to speak! Finding the balance is what we call being released—just enough muscular effort to speak, without so much that it impedes the function or freedom of the voice.

GOING INWARD: FINDING FREEDOM

Take some time now to sit quietly and reflect on a time that you felt physically free.
What are your own words for the sensation(s) of freedom?

_____

_____

_____

_____

_____

What parts of your body do you feel hold the most tension?

_____

_____

_____

_____

_____

Can you relate any of this tension to particular emotions or responses to stress?

_____

_____

_____

_____

_____

Can you remember a time before this tension pattern existed?

_____

_____

_____

_____

_____

Take yourself to a place with a mirror where you will not be disturbed. Bring a hand mirror so you can see yourself from the profile position. Look with kind eyes at your posture, from the front and the side. Notice the way your head sits atop your spine and the angle of your chin. What do you need to shift in order to move toward an anatomically neutral position? How does it feel to adjust your head this way?

_____

_____

_____

_____

_____

Make some notes here and/or draw a little or paste in a photo!

ALEXANDER TECHNIQUE

The first concept in finding freedom that made a lasting impression on me can be found within the Alexander technique. Frederick Matthias Alexander (1869–1955) was a professional actor who encountered hoarseness in his speech and eventually lost his voice completely. Even after resting his voice for two weeks he had major problems and could not work. The doctors he saw had no explanation for his vocal problems. From careful self-study he concluded that it was his posture and breathing habits when performing or projecting his voice that caused the problem. He noticed that he retracted his head, shortening the cervical spine and depressing his larynx. He also tensed his legs and overarched his back, in effect doing a "backbend." The conclusion of his self-study was that this pattern was clearly causing the problems with his voice. From this conclusion he proceeded to create a personal practice to inhibit this tension response and return to a free physical posture.

Alexander began to train himself to relax his body, allow his head to nod forward enough to lengthen his neck and to pause before speaking for just enough time that he could redirect the tension in his body. This stop and think moment is very like the practice of mindfulness. Building awareness of our vocal habits and postural tendencies is vital for us to learn how to unravel them. After Alexander had learned to elongate his spine and release tension from his body, he was able to work again as an actor. Other actors began to see the change in his work and he began to teach them his methods. Ultimately, he set up a training school and now the Alexander technique is taught internationally and used by all types of performers and many individuals as a way to improve posture as well as voice and breath. Alexander technique is usually done in one-to-one sessions. It is a common technique for musicians, actors and dancers as well as anyone wanting to improve postural health. Many conservatory programs for music and performing arts will have a resident Alexander teacher working with the students.

What I love about this technique is the purity of concept: underneath our learned habits of tension there is a freedom and natural alignment which allows our voices and our bodies to express totally. The ability to pause and notice the transition or moment when we tense reminds me of *nirodhah* from the *Yoga Sutras of Patanjali*.[6] In particular, the following translations of *nirodhah*—control, regulation, channeling, mastery, integration, coordination, understanding, stilling, quieting, setting aside of—can be transferred to the process of physical tension inhibiting our voice. What causes these inhibitions, or tension patterns, is our social or emotional conditioning. Instead of allowing emotion to be expressed or felt in response to the moment, most of us have learned to repress our emotional energy. Each moment we repress or deny the truth of our feelings the body registers tension and creates a pattern to cope with that tension. This is how all of the emotional responses that we have experienced in the past culminate in our current posture.

Much like the idea of the *koshas*, or energetic layers that make up a human, when we begin to observe ourselves as we speak, we must peel back the layers that have created the habits we use.

Principles and exercises

It will take time for you to learn how to "think" these directions rather than trying to "do" them, especially if your primary practice has been physical asana. Notice how they are called directions, not instructions! If you have been accustomed to physical work that is based in visual esthetics, you will also need to unlearn your habit of fitting the body into socially constructed norms. This is a way for you to let your particular body find a sense of release. Release is a different sensation to engagement. It is the difference between the muscular engagement against gravity and the letting go into gravity or momentum. Let go of any goal. Let go of any idea of what is correct. Allow feeling to be separated from judgment so you can feel what is. Get out of your way. Work with one direction at a time. Add the next direction slowly, only when you have a feeling for the previous ones and you are able to hold these directions in your body cumulatively. Try memorizing these principles and repeating them to yourself throughout the day, like you would a mantra.

Alexander's directions

1. *Let the neck be free*: Standing tall allows the muscles at the back of your head to relax. As this happens your chin will naturally drop slightly forward as the skull pivots down from the force of gravity. Take some time to feel that the head is balanced over the center of the spine and over the center of the chest. Aim for the top of the spine to stay between the ears. As often as possible during the day notice your neck and without judgment allow the muscles at the back of the neck to relax. Notice the effect.

2. *Head goes forward and up*: Imagining a direction for the head helps the head to center and the neck to stay free. Think forward, up as you move and when you are still. Aim for the air above your head; as you think about this area your head will

naturally move upward at a slightly forward diagonal angle. Make no effort, as effort makes tension. Simply think about the direction and let it happen. Notice the effect.

3. *Back lengthens*: When sitting, pay attention to the sit bones reaching down and the head reaching forward and up. When standing, let the length of your back begin at the heels, so the whole back line of the body lengthens. Again, this is an exercise in imagining and letting yourself open to new sensations. It is not an effort; it is a letting go into a new way of occupying your body and feeling the space around you.

4. *Back widens*: Think of widening across the front of the chest, across the armpits, across the upper back. Now through the middle of the back, across the solar plexus, along your lumbar area, then the low belly. Imagine yourself continually getting wider. No effort, no actual "movement." Just imagining and feeling.

5. *Knees forward and away*: Think of the knees moving forward and away as you walk. Notice how this affects your spine and the freedom in your neck.

Repeat all of the directions together until they come more naturally.

Pro tip
When leading trainings and day-long intensives, take extra care with your own seated position. Alexander's directions are a great reminder when we are sitting, to look for a long, wide back and the feeling of freedom in the neck. I sit on a couple of bolsters, a stack of bricks or whatever it takes for me to keep my posture in check during long hours of teaching, which is when it can get easy to let gravity take over.

The following exercises are based on the Alexander technique.

Semi-supine position

This is very similar to constructive rest. It is for the same purpose: to give your system a chance to stop and rest. It is from the resting position that we are able to shift out of tension patterns, which is a process that often begins with noticing what these tension patterns are. Do not be alarmed or turned off by the feeling that your body gets "tenser" as you are in the position. Unwinding tension takes time and practice.

Lie down as in constructive rest, with one or two small books behind your head. Think of the five directions, using them to anchor your mind in the present moment. Make no effort to do anything other than allow gravity to take effect as you think the directions. Sense the points of contact you have with the ground. Feel the weight of your body, let it sink down. Give your weight to the floor, allow yourself to be fully supported. Aim for 10–15 minutes, but allow yourself to start with shorter time frames if that helps you get in the habit of practicing regularly.

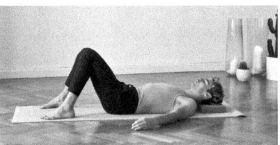

Crawling

Just like it sounds! Spend some time crawling on the floor to re-educate your muscles and coordination. Look down at the floor instead of forward, so the neck stays free and long. Make sure your knees are comfortable. Try it like a fly-girl and wear knee pads if needed! Think of Alexander's directions as you crawl. A few minutes is sufficient.

LINKLATER VOICE

Kristin Linklater was one of the most respected and prolific teachers of voice for actors. At 18 I was introduced to her methods in my voice classes at the University of California at Santa Barbara (UCSB). Her method is one of helping the speaker to know the workings of the body and find a deep connection to anatomical imagery. By using imagery of the body and then adding other types of imagery, we bypass our learned tension and emotional blocks. Like the Alexander technique, Linklater begins with a foundation of learning to relax.

> My approach to voice training is known as "freeing the natural voice"... The "freeing" part of it refers to letting go of habitual defensive tensions in the breathing and vocal tract musculature. The "natural" part refers to what is nature before nurture interferes. More than that, however, we can play with the idea that the organs of the body contain frequencies of sound—that the voice, indeed, already exists in the body waiting to be liberated. Mentally, there is a wonderful letting go of effort when one pictures the voice existing in vibrationary readiness in the organs, the pelvic basin, the hollows of the hip sockets, the thighs, the feet.[7]

The following exercises are based on Linklater's ideas.

The small "ff"

From a constructive rest or semi-supine position, become aware of your natural breathing rhythm.

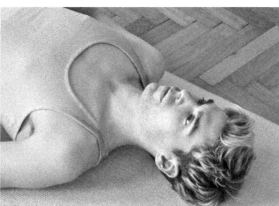

The long ha (1:2)

Inhale for the count of one, exhale for the count of two through the mouth making one long "haa" sound. Build up to higher counts, keeping the ratio, that is, 2:4, 6:12, etc. Do not force it or get to a place of feeling out of breath.

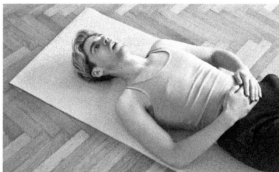

The little ha

With the same ratio of inhale/exhale as the long ha, make short "ha" sounds, repeating to the end of the exhale. Repeat while maintaining the feeling of an easy inhale.

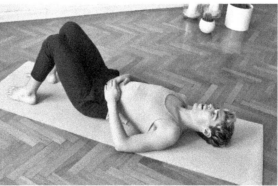

FITZMAURICE VOICEWORK©

Catherine Fitzmaurice studied at the Central School of Speech and Drama in London and after being introduced to Reichian psychology[8] and the therapy based on this work known as bioenergetics, she began to weave this work into her teaching. In 1968 she moved to the United States of America and studied yoga and shiatsu, which also began to influence her voice teaching. Currently (2019), Fitzmaurice Voicework represents the trend in theater and voice training toward blending Eastern and Western approaches. As with many other fields of personal development, bodywork and creative processes, we in the West are integrating Eastern practices more than ever before. I think this is one of the reasons that yoga has become so popular in the West; it is a part of this trend. This orientation toward looking at the actor/speaker/singer from a holistic point of view, taking into account the psycho-spirititual–emotional–energetic body, is what perhaps makes this method an easier access point for yoga teachers.

I spent over two years studying different forms of somatic practices, creative work and personal development at The Esalen Institute in Big Sur, California. During my time there I was lucky to be involved in bioenergetic therapy circles and movement workshops. I think this technique is unique in its definitive basis of *destructuring* and *restructuring* concepts. I have found that any training that I have participated in—whether for theater, dance, massage, movement or yoga—has had the effect of de-stabilizing my world view or my physical way of being. There is an accompanying discomfort, emotional chaos and often life-changing process to any worthwhile or deep learning experience.

In the Fitzmaurice work, the technique purposely takes students through a process known as *destructuring*, using physical and breath exercises to shift the practitioner out of set patterns of tension. This first phase is about exploring what is spontaneous, getting in touch with impulse and instinct. This is done with a sequence of physical positions that are a combination of yoga asana and adaptations of bioenergetics. These poses are not only held statically but done with equal focus on transitions, the poses leading to what Fitzmaurice calls "tremoring" or the release of energy in the body. From this release of energy, breathwork and sounding are introduced with the goal of the sound being a release of energy or flowing from the impulses of the body.

The next phase of *restructuring* encompasses reconnecting with the central nervous system (CNS) through specific muscular engagement of the deep abdominal and breathing muscles. This phase includes speaking as well as working with imagery akin to the Eastern energetic meridians and the philosophy of connecting lower body/mind with upper body/mind. For many students the process of destructuring, which can be applied conceptually to any learning or growth process, can be terrifying, perhaps to the point where fear stops the process. In this way, we are always in the process of learning. You may find that pausing at certain moments is necessary. Trusting that when we are ready the learning will continue is an important intention to hold during this process.

One of my theater teachers, Michael Morgan, describes the function of destructuring and restructuring in this way:

Since destructuring teaches the actor to honor the interior terrain of impulses, and experiential lessons bring to light the restrictive mechanisms of the past, the actor is primed to allow those insights to lead in the recovery of the functional self that operates in the outer world. The incitement is to maintain the spontaneity of the instincts—to retain a strong linkage to the autonomic nervous response system—while recovering the mental prowess of the central nervous system.[9]

I love this purposeful use of what many spiritual traditions recognize as walking through the fire or reaching our limit as a window into the next phase of development. If we want to make a change, we have to be willing to move through discomfort. It is not comfortable to release tension from the diaphragm, the jaw, the neck. There is a difference between physical discomfort and pain, and I never encourage pain in this or any physical work. I do, however, recognize and honor the important edge or awake quality that we feel in our body when the pose or the exercise is leading us toward something new.

Catherine Fitzmaurice's work has been an important example to me of effective ways of synthesizing Eastern practices with theater training and providing a framework for how to approach any training. I encourage you to seek out qualified teachers if this work calls to you, as well as incorporating the principles into any practice, whether yoga or voice. I will not present exercises directly from her work, yet I hope you will explore much of her theory within the following exercises.

BASIC WARM-UP TECHNIQUES

This is a collection of techniques that I have learned in many different types of acting classes over the years.

Sweet and sour

Facial stretches: pretend you ate a lemon and squeeze your face tight and small. Then pretend you ate a sweet. Open your face as big as possible! Repeat a few times.

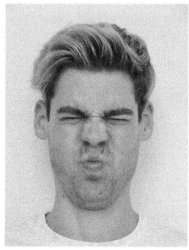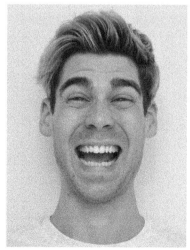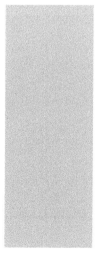

Pro tip
Yawn it out. I heard the legendary Morgan Freeman say in an interview that he thinks yawns are the best warm-up for the voice. Sneak in a yawn whenever you can to discreetly open the throat area and help your pitch stay optimal. When you can't do more of a warm-up, at the very least give yourself a big yawn.

Body rolls and undulation

From standing, find a steady breath. Imagine you are seaweed. Allow a wave to pulse through you from head toe. Exhale and roll down the spine like a moving forward fold, then bend the knees and roll back up with a strong impulse and a sense of rhythm. Do not go for precision of spinal rolls, go for a flowing movement that is breath initiated. This gets the blood pumping and helps release tension from the whole body. When possible have a friend spot you to help you flow through the whole body instead of moving mechanically.

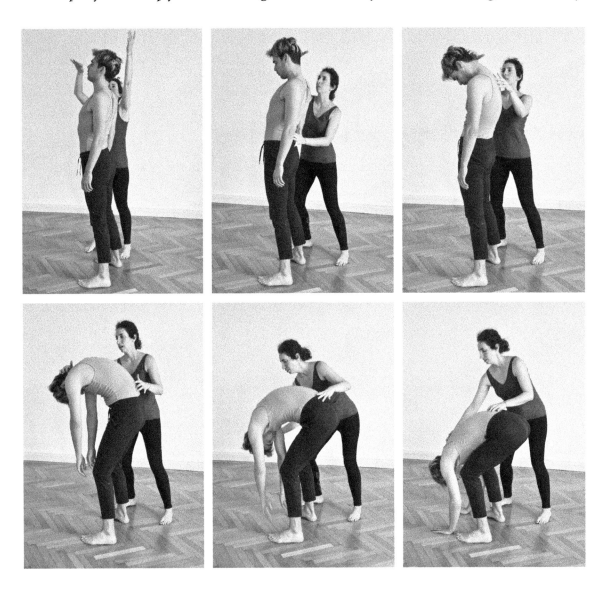

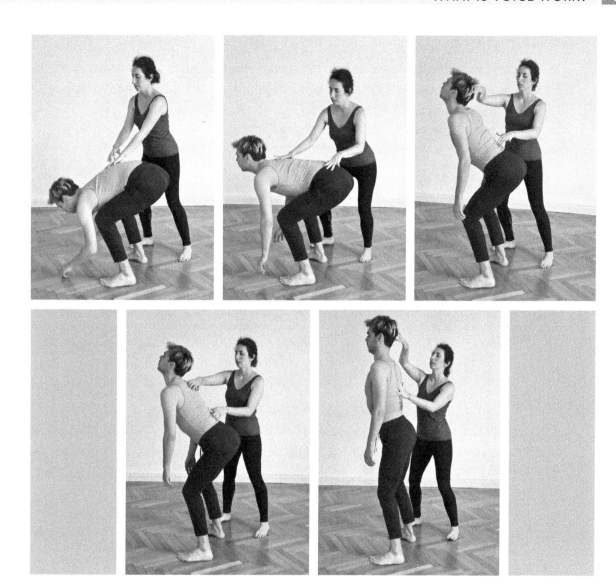

Helicopter arms swings

With open mouth and uncontrolled sound from the lowest area of your belly on an exhale, let the arms swing loose so they flap against the body.

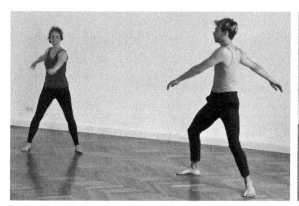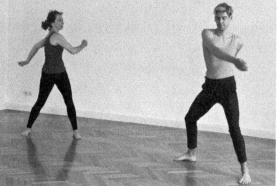

Arm swings with chi gong

With a loose fist continue swinging the arms with momentum. Have the loose fists hit to activate the upper chest (lung points) and the back just under the ribs (kidney points). On the exhale, when the fists make contact with the body, exhale with the sound "shew."

 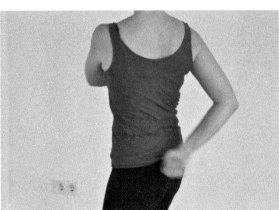 

Joyous arm swings

This builds on what you have been doing but now includes bending the knees and letting the arms swing all the way up. This often creates an uplifting mood and a sense of readiness. It's a great one if you only have time for one warm-up. Notice how when the arms move upward the voice also rises in pitch.

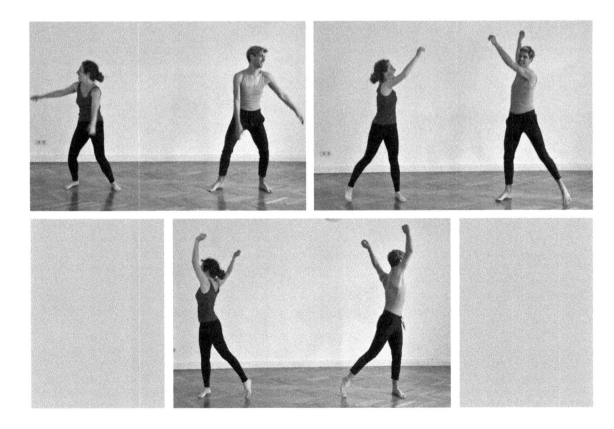

Self-massage

Touch is a great way to release tension, and self-massage is free and easy. Start by working on your shoulders if this area is most familiar to you for receiving massage. Knead the trapezius as firmly as possible without creating pain. Be gentle as you work on the neck and avoid the front of the throat for now. With clean hands reach your first two fingers into the mouth and use your thumb on the outside of the cheek. Reaching toward the back of the jaw, find the muscle in the cheek—it is usually like a small button. Press gently with thumb and fingers to work the muscle.

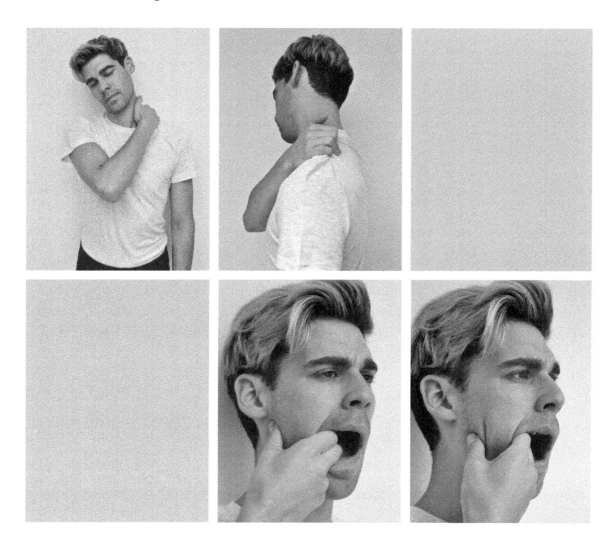

Voice box massage

With a gentle hold on your Adam's apple, swallow a few times while giving light pressure through your fingers. Then make small circles around it, and while humming give a small rocking motion, moving your fingers up and down the front of the throat. Use only a light, gentle touch on this delicate area of your body.

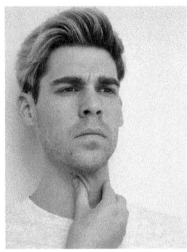

Scalene/front of throat

Again, use only light pressure and awareness that this area is very fragile. With an open hand give even, light pressure along the front of the neck as you let your head rest toward the other shoulder. This is a combination of stretching with massage. Do not force anything or work aggressively. Small and often is much better than working deeply.

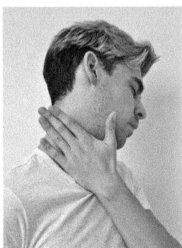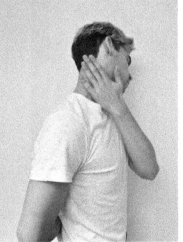

Neck stretch

Assist the stretch with very gentle pressure from the top hand and arm. Doing this often enough that you begin to enjoy letting the top arm rest passively on the head is a great goal for increasing elasticity in one of the areas that for most of us is tight and restricted.

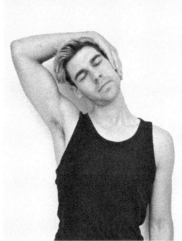

Jaw massage

Dig your fingertips into the grooves at the back of your jaw where it hinges (see the diagram). Make circles along the jaw muscles. Open and close the jaw while giving pressure. Get into the areas that are tight respectfully. Again, avoid going too deeply too quickly and make this a regular practice rather than a strong one.

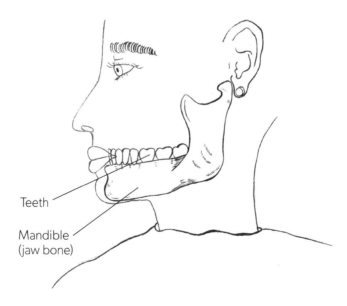

Teeth

Mandible
(jaw bone)

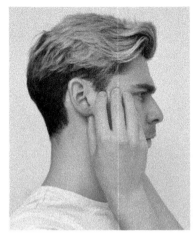 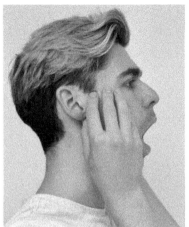 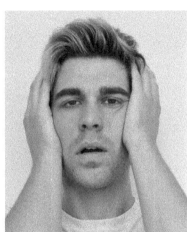

Jaw release

This is one of my all-time favorites. It has a tendency to make us giggle, because it involves funny and involuntary sounds. However, if you are laughing or smiling the tension in your face will block the exercise from being effective. So, laugh it out first and when you are able to proceed without a tense face give it a try.

Clasp your hands firmly together, interlacing your fingers fully. Hold the hands in front of your chest with bent elbows. Relax your face until your jaw hangs open. As you exhale with *sound* begin to shake your arms so vigorously that your jaw flaps up and down. Let the flapping continue as you exhale with sound, so the combination of flapping and sound vibration creates a full release for your jaw and throat. Enjoy the funny sounds that will escape as you allow them to come forth unrestrained by judgments.

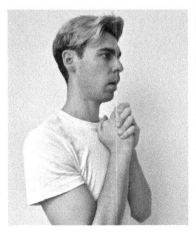 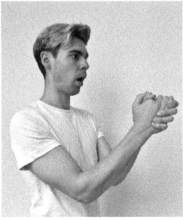 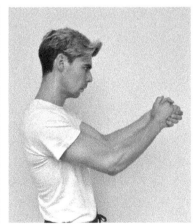

Pelvic power

Start in a low setu bandhasana (bridge pose) with your arms outstretched comfortably. Try different arm variations to find what is best for you to feel free in your throat. On the inhale, lower the pelvis only a couple of centimeters. As you exhale make the sound "ha" and lift the pelvis back up. Find a bouncing rhythm for your pelvis and sound to come together. Try different speeds; notice how the sound changes in volume and pitch. Try circles, figure of eights and free movement of your pelvis combined with exhale and sound. Shaking and rocking in rhythm with your breath can also be done in this shape to help you free your voice.

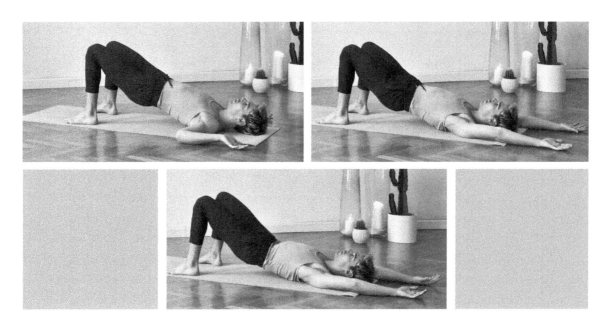

The following "Pitch" and "Resonance work" sections are based on my notes from "Voice for actors" with Judith Olauson at UCSB.

PITCH

We all have a habitual pitch, the way we normally speak. Pitch is registered as high or low, and we know that a lower pitch is generally preferred by all listeners. The pitch you use in daily life might not work for teaching. This is where we work to find your optimum pitch. Our culture favors lower pitches, but if our pitch is too low, it can be harder to project and can also strain the voice. Everyone has an optimum pitch and we can all find it; it is sometimes called our middle range. Every voice has a range, some more varied than others. Being able to go up and down the scale of your range should be done playfully and after warming up. Doing this work is the way to find and become familiar with using it. If it's hard for you to find your voice going higher or lower, please consider working with a voice coach. Speaking from the optimal pitch, or pitches close to it, will help your voice to be stronger and clearer. When you know your middle range try starting a sentence from a slightly higher pitch than you normally use. This is because most intonation drops lower through a sentence and when you start a little bit higher, you then have room to move into a lower pitch without getting out of your midrange low.

Exercise: finding optimum pitch

Place your hand on your Adam's apple and say EEEEEE in your highest voice, really extending the sound with an exaggerated length. Then on the same exhale say OOOOH in your lowest voice, again extending the sound. Feel how the larynx moves positions in the throat as you change from a high to low sound. Now begin with a low OOOOH and slowly begin to change the sound toward your higher position. Go very slowly and make sure there is never a strain on your vocal cords. Do this again, opening the sound from OOOOH to UHHH with no strain. Notice where you feel most comfortable making this open UHHH sound. Speak on that tone; that is your optimal pitch level. Do this exercise as part of your vocal routine and begin to strengthen your ability to make comfortable and strong sounds on either side of your optimal pitch level so that you expand your vocal palette.

RESONANCE WORK

Remember that literal resonance is how our voice is enlarged or amplified, and the areas that we use help determine the quality of the sound. The following exercises are meant to create more balance and correct the over- or underuse of certain resonators.

Use the following techniques with the sentence "Mary had a little lamb."

Pharyngeal resonance

Focus your voice toward the back of the mouth and say AH while laying fingers on the outside of the upper throat so that you can feel a strong vibration. Say the sentence, maintaining the vibration in the upper throat and very little vibration from the mouth or nasal cavities. Open the mouth widely and keep your pitch low.

Oral resonance

Close your lips and puff out your cheeks, and bring your focus to the mouth and not the throat. Place your fingers gently on your cheeks and prolong the EE sound to feel the vibration in the mouth on your fingertips. Use as little pharyngeal or nasal resonance as possible; keep it in the mouth and cheeks. Overwork the lips with each word.

Nasal resonance

Start by humming an NG sound and sustaining it to feel the vibration along the nose and the fingers on either side of your nose. Sense the downward relaxed position at the back of your soft palate as you do this. Now shift between the NG sound and the AAH sound (as in the word "fat") to feel your palate moving up and down. When the palate is in the down position, most of the air comes out the nose. Say the sentence, trying to nasalize as many sounds as possible. Keep the pitch low to help feel this exaggerated nasal resonance.

Getting to know your resonators

To hear and feel more nasal resonance say the following:

Many men and women are under tension in modern America.

Modern Millie demanded remuneration commensurate with male employees in similar management positions.

Flinging the gauntlet once indicated wanting to engage in a duel.

My mama makes me mad whenever she remembers and recounts the many mischievous misadventures of my immature adolescence.

Oral and pharyngeal sounds—focus on an open throat as you say:

Fight the good fight fearlessly.

She freely spiced the rice with herbs or flavor additives.

Whittle twigs of teak wood as well as oak, acacia or poplar trees.

Take daily walks beside the big skyscrapers at Wall Street.

I hope you will be able to assist Betty Baker with her project for the physics laboratory.

Theodore thought that thistles were a cactus species, but they are just prickly bush.

VOCAL HEALTH KNOW-HOW

Whenever I have to teach for long hours on a training or if I am starting to feel sick, I must stick to a very healthy regime. I consider the quality of the air where I am teaching. In cold months teaching with the heaters running full blast makes the air so dry that I have lost my voice when leading a weekend training. The next time I taught in that room I put wet towels on the radiators to put some moisture back in the air. It helped a lot. When actors are in a show, especially for extended runs and double bills, they will often not speak when they are off stage. We call this vocal rest. It is really important to consider when you are traveling as a visiting teacher, leading trainings and teaching form over three hours a day. Serious actors will also put their vocal health ahead of their socializing if they want to be onstage with an effective voice. One way that I remind myself to keep my talking to a minimum when I am teaching a lot or feeling weak is to wear a scarf, even indoors. It keeps my throat warm and is a physical reminder of my priority.

Rules for a healthy voice

- No smoking.

- Avoid caffeine and alcoholic drinks—they dehydrate vocal folds and make the mucus membrane vulnerable!

- Moisturize your vocal folds with steam inhalations.

- Drink plenty of water.

- Lessen acid reflux, sometimes brought on by food or lack of sleep and stress.

- Avoid milk products—they create mucus on the vocal folds.

- Keep your head straight when talking, especially on the phone.

- Keep your abdomen free to move—avoid tight belts and restrictive clothes.

- Instead of coughing to clear your throat, pause for a deep breath, swallow and take water or tea—coughing or "clearing the throat" presses the folds too strongly and also dries them out. If you must cough or clear the throat, do it gently.

- Get plenty of sleep—the voice registers even a small degree of tiredness.

- Keep your mouth closed and breathe through your nose when out in cold and damp weather.

- Avoid talking when you are tired, your throat is dry or if you are hungry.

- When under emotional strain, talk less.

- Avoid long talks when drinking alcohol—the larynx becomes desensitized and you are apt to misuse your voice.

- Use lozenges and sprays for your throat only when you are actually sick—they also desensitize the larynx.

- When you have to talk above a constant or background noise, try to rest your voice as often as possible to counteract the strain.

- Use restorative practices to help avoid burnout.

Benefits and goals of working on your voice

- Release of the neck, larynx, bottom of the mouth, jaw muscles.

- Improvement of the flexibility of the larynx.

- Improvement of the vocal sound.

- A larger vocal range.

- Reduction of the feeling of having something stuck in one's throat or other complaints of tension.

- Reduction of instances where the voice gets "lost" or hoarse.

DIET AND LIFESTYLE: EASTERN TRADITIONAL MEDICINES FOR VOCAL HEALTH

Ayurveda can be used to help you find a healthier vocal routine. I also consider traditional Chinese medicine in how I eat and plan my days. If I want my voice to be at its best I avoid "cooling" foods and aim for "warming" foods that are low in white sugar, cooked vegetables over raw foods and broths over creamed soups. I don't eat right before teaching, if possible. Drinking something warming is a good habit to be in, before teaching and also during class. I am not a nutritionist so I would encourage you to consult specialists or books that inspire you to look at the food you eat through the lens of taking care of your voice.

My favorite tea for throat comfort is a combination of fresh ginger, fresh mint, whole cloves and cinnamon sticks brewed together. YUM. The following are other great teas and infusions to drink at a warm or hot temperature:

- green tea

- oolong teas

- turmeric

- cinnamon

- ginger (excellent to prevent sore throat and clear the voice).

These are great foods to include in your diet:

- dark leafy greens (spinach, collard greens, kale, Swiss chard)

- broccoli

- carrots

- raspberries

- blueberries

- strawberries

- grapes

- cherries.

Neti pot

A great way to keep your resonators clear and keep mucus to a minimum is regular use of the neti pot. This is a common kriya, or cleansing practice from the tradition of Ayurveda. My first time with a neti pot was in my initial teacher training in Los Angeles with Ana Forrest. There were about 40 of us on the training all doing neti pot with bowls of water and towels in the yoga room. Laughing actually helped the water go up our noses. It's best to use a saline solution that is made for this practice as well as distilled or boiled water. Getting the ratio of salt to water right is important so that it doesn't give you a burning sensation. Tilting your head at an angle that helps gravity move the water is sometimes tricky. Take your time. I do not recommend this when you have an acute sinus infection as it can push the infection deeper into the sinuses. Regular practice of neti pot will hopefully keep you clearer and less susceptible to head colds.

 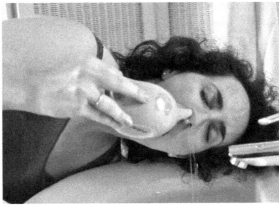 

Pro tip
Traveling teachers are constantly under the stress of flying, which is brutal on the voice as well as the sinuses, and in general makes us tired and more susceptible to illness. Regular neti pot before, during and after traveling is a great way to stay healthier. Take vocal rest seriously; I know a lot of teachers who lose their voices when leading trainings, intensives and retreats. If you have to speak for more than three hours at a time, be sure to build into your day plenty of time that you are *not* talking at all and doing restorative practice.

3

SPEAKING YOUR TRUTH

Once more; speak clearly, if you speak at all;
Carve every word before you let it fall;
Don't, like a lecturer or dramatic star,
Try over hard to roll the British R;
Do put your accents in the proper spot;
Don't, —let me beg you, —don't say "How?" for "What?"
And, when you stick conversation's burrs,
Don't strew your pathway with those dreadful urs.

Oliver Wendell Holmes (1846)
Urania: A Rhymed Lesson. Boston: William D. Ticknor & Company (p.22)

During a recent 200-hour yoga teacher training, I worked with students who were asked to brainstorm the kinds of verbal cues that work best for them. I think this is a great way to find the cues and the type of teaching language you want to use. Here are some findings that are helpful to keep in mind when you teach: clarity, pace of speaking matching the pace of the practice, details, encouraging tone of voice, using the voice to bring the class energy up or relax the room, softer voice during challenging poses, energizing voice during challenging poses, allowing personality and humor to come through, telling stories and weaving in philosophy. On the flip side, when asked what didn't work well, these responses stood out: too much personal information or joking, strict or dry attitude, childish words and imagery that doesn't make sense or is vague. Notice that with any of these it comes down to an opinion of the student; to one person it could be that the story was too personal and to another not.

Let's break these ideas down and explore what it really means to use them in our teaching in terms of voice.

CLARITY

This is a combination of speaking clearly (enunciation, articulation) so that people can literally understand the words you are saying. This is sometimes called diction; however, the definition of diction is the choice and use of words in speaking as well as the way you speak. Everyone has a unique way of speaking, similar to the voiceprint that is based on our genetic code, which is influenced by where we have lived and the people we grew up around. Our environment is a huge factor in how we speak. Without abandoning your way of speaking entirely you can work on improving your skills.

Enunciation and articulation

One of the most effective ways to practice articulation is to work with tongue twisters and to over-enunciate or completely exaggerate the way you are saying words. This builds elasticity in the mouth and face, which is the opposite of holding tension and will lead to your voice coming out more clearly. These exercises use repetition, which is important for training your mouth to articulate.

Articulation is shaping the sounds using your articulators—your tongue and the way it touches your teeth, for example. Consonants are the best for finding strong articulation. Consonants stop or control the flow of air and sound. They have less carrying power, so the voice is not projected as easily on the consonant part of the sound. Consonants are the parts of the word that make words understood by giving precision to what you say. Some consonant sounds are unvoiced in regular speech. This can create a lazy mouth, where consonants that should be voiced, or heard, can be lost. Most articulation problems regarding clarity come from issues with consonant sounds. If you notice that you mumble or do not allow your mouth to open enough for the sounds to come out clearly, try doing tongue twisters and the following exercises with a small cork between your teeth. Take a cork from a bottle and cut it to a comfortable size that you can practice with.

Exercises

Practice the following while embracing silliness and exaggerating the movement of your tongue. Remember, this is an exercise that will lead to the words sounding clearer when you speak normally. It is like a warm-up for a bigger yoga pose, a component part that you need to prepare for the peak pose. Take the time to warm up first, using the exercises from Chapter 2 that give you the most released upper body and openness through the throat, so that as you play you can keep the vocal cords from being strained. I recommend the Alexander technique-inspired work as well as the breathing with released voice from the Linklater technique.

Here is a classic exercise used in drama warm-ups across the English-speaking world. In some drama classes we were asked to recite this while doing jumping jacks!

What a to-do to die today, at a minute or two to two;
a thing distinctly hard to say, but harder still to do.
For they'll beat a tattoo, at a quarter to two
with a rat-tat-tat- tat-tat-tat- tat-tat-tattoo

and the dragon will come when he hears the drum
at a minute or two to two today, at a minute or two to two.

Here are some shorter ones to practice with—after over-enunciating, try them as fast as possible while pronouncing each word correctly and clearly:

The perfectly purple bird unfurled its curled wings and whirled over the world.

The weary wanderer wondered wistfully whether winsome Winifred would weep.

The queen was a coquette.

They know not whence, nor whither, where nor why.

The very merry Mary crossed the ferry in a fur coat.

Shouldn't, wouldn't, couldn't.

Round the rugged rock, the little letter grieved, sagged and sighed.

Many anemones see an enemy anemone.

Repeat over and over, seeing how fast and clear you can be:

It takes time to untangle 22 tutus.

She sells seashells by the seashore.

Rubber baby buggy bumpers.

Red leather, yellow leather.

Eleven benevolent elephants.

Vowel play

The vowel sounds are the parts of the word that best express the emotion of the speaker. They also carry the voice best and are easiest to use for projecting sound. All vowel sounds are voiced, unless you are whispering. Vowels require the whole mouth to move in a different way from consonants. Vowels are identified by their pitch, resonance and how long they are pronounced for.

Mispronunciation and "accents"

Everyone has an accent. You don't generally hear your own accent because you are used to it, you grew up with other people speaking similarly and your ear is not as sensitive to the sounds you are familiar with. Whatever your accent is, speaking clearly is not the same as trying to lose an accent. Your accent is part of you, and teaching authentically requires you to embrace all parts of yourself. It's important to notice that if you are teaching a population of students who have a different accent to yours, that can be a block to them understanding you easily. When I am in this situation, which I have been in now for over a decade, I will ask someone in the room to give me a local pronunciation. This is the kind of moment that often breaks the ice and helps the room feel friendlier. If teaching in a country with a different native language (and not using a translator), you can always ask students in the room to help out with words that might be less familiar. I found a lot of students in Austria don't know the English word knuckle, so when I instruct cues about the knuckles in *hasta bandha* (hand seal, or engagement of the hands on the mat) I often ask someone to say it for me in German.

In a lot of my workshops I meet students who are teaching in a language that is not their mother tongue. Mastering a new language is hard enough, so if you are working in English (for one example) but not speaking it regularly, this will show up in your pronunciation. Pronunciation is the combination of our hearing—how we hear the word—and our ability to make the sounds clearly. Listening and repeating exercises are most helpful for improving pronunciation. If you are serious about working on this, take the time to listen to a speech before speaking it back. Record this process and listen back to check if you are making the sounds similarly or where you can improve. If specific sounds are hard for you to master, use the tongue twisters that include those sounds and practice them with recording. When I was a young student in Spain I worked as a pronunciation coach for someone taking an oral exam in English for her law degree. We would meet to converse and I would stop her and make her repeat words that were not easy for her, until they became easier. I also made her tapes to listen to and repeat on her own. Finding someone who can help you in this way is very important, as sometimes we are not the best at listening to ourselves!

The way we mispronounce words or say them in a way that is hard to understand is often through the following: omission (dropping a sound), substitution, switching sounds, adding sounds, and transposing or misplacing the accent/stress on the wrong syllable. Accent/stress is where you place most force on your word, the syllable that has most stress. Whenever you aren't sure of correct pronunciation take the time to look it up in the dictionary and notice the diacritical markings and accents, or use the sound option and listen to the computer voice. Personally, I think it's a valuable skill to be able to read the diacritical markings and to know which syllable should be stressed. But hey, I'm a lover of language and a theater nerd used to marking scripts. Here is a list of words you can practice saying out loud. Try saying these words clearly and notice if you have any habits of dropping or adding sounds.

Words with sounds commonly omitted:

adjective

company

environment

February

government

literature

poem

recognize

understanding.

Words with sounds commonly substituted:

absurd

chimney

diphtheria

genuine

heroism

Italian

partner

pronunciation

sandwich

welts.

Words with sounds commonly added:

accompanist

brethren

burglar

disastrous

escape

height

positively

tremendous

umbrella

Washington.

Words with sounds often transposed:

aggravate

cavalry

children

introduction

larynx

modern

perspiration

pretty

professor

secretary.

Words with often misplaced syllabic stress:

ascertain

deluge

executor

formidable

guitar

infamous

maintenance

mischievous

police

theater.

PACING

The pace of our words is often a window into our internal state. Anxiety and nerves tend to speed people up. They can also go the other way and freeze us. Figuring out your tendency is part of this process. It's another reason that listening to yourself teaching can be so illuminating. You can actually measure what is called your *speech rate*, which is calculated as your number of words spoken in a minute (wpm). Famous politicians and speakers usually have one commonality for their speech rates: they mix it up. Professional speakers know how to slow down or speed up their pace of speech to create the effect they want. In general, the more slowly we speak, the more importance our words seem to hold. Slower speech is recommended for introducing new ideas and imparting serious information. Faster speech is heard as passionate, exciting, motivating and often emotional. When we speak quickly it can grab an audience's attention, yet if we keep that pace it becomes overwhelming and confusing. You can use your pacing to build energy in a strong flow, and then to slow down your speaking pace as you hold a pose or release it. To get a sense of the importance of timing I recommend listening to great speakers. Try these to start: Martin Luther King Jr., Barack Obama, Amy Tan, Oprah Winfrey. TED talks are a great way to notice the effect of pacing during speaking.

Exercise for tempo variation

Play with the following phrases by changing speed to notice how that affects the meaning of what is being said. Observe and give ample time to breath pauses.

(Faster tempo) *We should have a great many fewer disputes in the world if words were taken for what they are—*(slower) *the signs of our ideas only, and not for things themselves.*

Now reverse the tempos to see the difference. You can play this game with many small speeches that you enjoy. You can also play this game with your teaching instruction, reading from the sutras or any text that inspires you.

MODULATION

Modulation refers to the way we vary the strength, tone and pitch of our voice. It is similar to inflection, or the rise and fall of the tone of voice within a word or sentence. Modulation is key in using your voice as a tool for teaching. The number one complaint I hear in all of my workshops is about the dreaded "yoga teacher voice," which tends to be monotone. Breaking out of this trap is done with practice; reading this book and doing the exercises will help ensure you don't fall into the trap. Monotone speaking puts people to sleep. My favorite example of monotone speaking is the part of the movie *Ferris Bueller's Day Off* when the teacher is taking roll and calling out names. He says each name with the same exact tone, making the names meaningless, as the camera shows the boredom on the faces of the students. If you want to disengage people or prove something boring, use a monotone voice.

If you want to inspire people, introduce ideas, reach people and communicate, then your voice must be colorful. It must move all around in a natural way. If you normally speak in one register, this is a growing edge to find and play with, making your voice more flexible. Your voice also helps modulate the energy in the room. For instance, when teaching inversions or back bends often the students become overexcited and the room can get chatty. When this is happening, can you use a bell to quiet the room and then a soft and commanding voice to move them into the next pose? Sometimes we need a softer voice to help bring us down to earth, rather than another energizing element.

Another example of using a voice that is less expected, or is not prescriptive, is when students are in a challenging pose, maybe a balancing pose or one that requires a lot of focus. Even though this might be the peak of the class or an instance when you want the student to be fully engaged, using a softer voice can actually be helpful. The change of tone can grab attention and help people hear you and focus. I find the softer voice is most effective when next to a louder moment, so that in the ensuing silence they are able to breathe and listen more deeply. It is not only the soft quality and low volume that can be a surprise that will make students' ears prick up, it is also slowing down the vowels and extending the length of your words.

Radio and television broadcasters classically modulate their voices to have a lower pitch and put stresses on words that create an unnatural rhythm of speaking. As a game you can do a news version of any text to play with having a lower pitch and putting an extra punch on certain words. Listen to an announcer you enjoy or one who makes you laugh and spend some time imitating their way of speaking. Remember, being playful is the most effective way to create new pathways in your brain. Perhaps find a friend to play this game with.

Another game for increasing your ability to use inflection is to reverse what you normally do. Speak a portion of any text (pick up a newspaper and read it out loud into a recorder) and notice your inflection—where does your voice go, up or down? Where do you stress each word? Which word in the sentence is stressed most? Then, reverse what you have done. Try going down in pitch on the words or parts of the words that you previously went up on. Remember that this is a technical exercise meant to teach your voice it can break free of habit. Keep it playful. Start any of these playful exercises with at least ten minutes of the relaxation and breath exercises from Chapters 1 and 2. Warming up is key to keeping these exercises healthy for the voice.

Pitch power in contrasts

Practice these sentences out loud to feel the change in pitch and meaning. Remember that the way you speak should back up what you say, and when it doesn't the dissonance can be felt by whomever you are speaking to:

The sun is rising. Is the sun rising?

Is she coming home? She is coming home.

The coffee is ready. Is the coffee ready?

Did you let the cat out? You let the cat out.

Your homework is done. Is your homework done?

Can you swim? You can swim.

She has written you a letter. Has she written you a letter?

Can he play piano? He can play piano.

They have just moved into the house. Have they just moved into the house?

Intonation = truth

Every language has a musical quality to it, which comes from the rise and fall of inflection as we speak. English has a lot of opportunities for pitch changes and a lot of words that mean completely different things depending on the way you use your intonation. Here are some guidelines to be aware of in your speech and those around you:

- A higher pitch on a single word is a way of getting attention or interrupting a conversation.

- Changes in pitch allow people to hear how the speaker is feeling.

- Pitch change mostly occurs on the stressed syllable of the word.

- Pitch change is often on the most important word in the sentence or phrase.

- Pitch change occurs at the end of the message to signify the speaker is finished. This is generally a lower pitch.

- Teachers should be sensitive to the multiple ways in which students will interpret what the teacher says and take account not only of what they say but the way they say it. Notice if your accent includes any pitch change habits that could confuse your meaning. For example, if you typically raise your pitch at the end of a sentence it can be interpreted as a question when you might be making a statement.

VOCAL STYLINGS FOR YOGA TEACHING

When teaching in a class environment for yoga we generally need three specific styles of voice projection and tone. In no prioritized order, these are: energizing, relaxing, individual. We need our instruction to at times energize, motivate or enthuse our students. At other moments we need to bring the energy down or relax the students into a calmer attitude. At many times we need to address an individual in front of the whole group, while making it clear that an instruction is just for one.

This is something I work with teachers on individually, in person or online. What is hardest for most people, including experienced teachers, is using a relaxing tone of voice while projecting the voice loudly enough that everyone can hear. I find a quiet voice that I cannot understand or hear the opposite of relaxing. The trick is to remember your vowel play. Lengthen your vowels so that your voice is carried further and is more able to impart the emotion you want. Avoid whispering or singsong speech.

Encouraging the group requires full projection and also a strong belief that what you are saying is important. It requires us to have a sense of leading, being in charge of the room. The emotional work required for this is found in all of our *Going inward* reflective prompts. If you don't believe that the students want to hear you, if your imposter's syndrome or whatever critical voice in your head is still blocking you, go back to your personal work. Realistically, this work is never-ending. Often when we think something is resolved it can come back in a different or similar form. Many teachers who struggle with this type of speaking are still hiding, not comfortable being seen or taking charge. Be gentle with yourself if this is a challenge.

Addressing one student in a group of many is easiest when you know their name or can at least make eye contact. Students might be focusing on something completely different, so being clear that the cue is for them can be portrayed with your voice. Of course, the instruction is not private and in fact many other students might benefit from the cue. We do as teachers need to be able to single someone out (hopefully with an encouraging voice and positive way of directing their attention), which you can practice as well.

Exercise

Make sure you have warmed up your voice properly. Start with the pelvic power exercise in Chapter 2, and add some of the resonance exercises from earlier in this chapter and any other poses or practices that give you an embodied vocal connection.

Now set a recorder or a friend on the other side of the room. In your mind identify which voice you are going to practice first, second and third. If you are working with a friend, don't tell them your order! Do explain these three types of voice. Using a line or sentence from a nursery rhyme or poem you learned as a child (something you know by heart in your mother tongue), deliver the line in each vocal style and then listen to see if you can tell the difference or ask your friend. This will show you clearly if you are communicating what you intend to as well as if you are loud enough. Another way to do this is with video, so that you can look at your body language as well, which we will get into in the next chapter.

Whether we like a voice or not is purely subjective but it can be looked at more analytically. As you identify which actors', speakers' and teachers' voices you enjoy listening to or don't, take a moment to use the voice and diction evaluation form below as a way to evaluate your preferences. Start with a sample from someone else before you venture to chart yourself. Ultimately, this can also help you to identify your own voice, as listening to yourself and (as objectively as possible) charting your vocal traits will help you describe your natural tendencies with more precision than just good or bad. It might also lead you to identify which exercises will help you most (e.g. if you find your voice really nasal, then choose the voice work to help you use other resonators in more balance). Notice that this is only to be done long after you have worked with the self-reflection and empowerment work from Chapter 1! If this brings you down, skip it until you have a stronger day and feel more objective.

Voice and diction evaluation form[10]

Mark each category as: Very good, Average, Unsatisfactory

Rate
Too fast
Too slow
Unvarying, monotonous
Poor phrasing
Irregular rhythm of speaking
Hesitations
Repeated word crutches

Loudness
Too loud
Too weak
Lack of variety, monotony
Force overused as a form of emphasis

Pitch
General level too high
General level too low
Lack of variety, monotony
Fixed pattern, predictable
Exaggerated pitch changes

Quality
Nasal
Denasal
Hoarse, husky
Breathy
Throaty, harsh
Strained, strident, shrill
Flat, lack of vibrato
Falsetto
Tremorous

Diction
Speech sounds complete
Indistinct articulation, oral inactivity
Slow, labored
Rapid, slurring
Mispronunciation

General impressions
Favorable:
Friendliness
Alertness
Self-assurance
Vitality
Poise
Responsiveness

Unfavorable:
Indifference
Timidity
Tenseness
Indecision
Unfriendliness
Affectation
Unresponsiveness
Immaturity

LANGUAGE

The words we use when teaching communicate to our students more than simply how to get in and out of poses. I believe that language is extremely important and that it contributes to the attitude we impart to our students as well as any hierarchy in the room. In Chapter 7 I will introduce you to *nonviolent communication* (NVC), the work of Dr. Marshal B. Rosenberg, a technique that has revolutionized the way I communicate and continues to teach me as I learn to practice it. In this section we are focusing on cues for getting students to work within a pose, as well as how to essentialize the instructional element or "how to" we are directing. In some yoga lineages there are teaching scripts that must be adhered to. Personally, I cannot understand how teaching from a script would be fulfilling after any length of time. I do see how novices can feel safe when there is a script to rely on. I am hoping that those of you using this book are working off script, as in choosing your own words. If not, perhaps this chapter will help you learn how to find your own words. Our creative work—the product, if you will—as yoga teachers is our language. It is what we say to put our individual approach into a package that our students understand.

Active verbs

A quick and effective technique for your teaching language is to know when you are using active versus passive verbs. For a dynamic class, active verbs are the best way to get people to embody actions and movements. These are the verbs that end with *ing*. We want to instruct the pose as something that one is doing, which continues to emphasize autonomy. Passive verbs are more effective when teaching observation, mindfulness or restorative poses in which the focus is on feeling and witnessing the fluctuations of mind and body.

When we begin teaching, we will often parrot or mimic the words of our teachers. There is nothing wrong with this; if the words speak to you and resonate deeply then there will be a genuine delivery. If, however, you don't really resonate with the words, they will sound affected or removed. They will not land or be understood by your audience. The power of your words comes from your own conviction. At some point in your teaching you will find your own spin on things, and that is what makes your teaching interesting and personal. When you want to expand your vocabulary, start with the typical words that we need as yoga teachers.

GOING INWARD: EXPANDING YOUR VOCABULARY

How many ways can you say "lengthen"? Here are my examples:

- elongate

- extend

- reach

- expand upward

- move up

- create space

- feel gently pulled up

- stretch

- draw up.

_____

_____

_____

How can you describe "breathing"?

_____

_____

_____

How many ways can you say "stabilize"?

_____

_____

_____

How many ways can you say "quiet"?

_____

_____

_____

How many ways can you describe a direction (e.g. up, down, in, out, right, left)?

_____

_____

_____

Notice other actions or themes that you hear in classes or feel in your own practice. Make more lists that help expand your vocabulary for teaching. Move into metaphor, simile and analogy. Try to find these for any pose you are focusing on. For example, if your peak pose is urdhva dhanurasana, you can make a flow chart starting with free association. Not only for peak poses, but for any pose you spend time instructing you will want to have more than less to say. As teachers when we are passionate about our subject and when we have a deep grasp of it, we should be in the mode of editing ourselves when we teach. The longer I teach, the more I continue to peel back the unnecessary or less effective words and anecdotes.

Here is an example of a simple free association for a peak pose:

Upward facing bow

Bow. Tension. Where is the tension in a bow? Where in this pose are we engaged? Engagement. How we engage with the world, how we face things, how much energy we bring to what we are doing…

Where do we overwork?

What might we learn from our life in how we approach this pose?

Do we overwork in general?

When have I personally overworked myself? Do I have an appropriate story that can help people see the connection between this physical asana and our attitude toward life?

Try a few yourself!

Pose:

_____

_____

_____

_____

_____

Pose:

_____

_____

_____

_____

_____

Metaphors and similes

Take the previous lists you made of words and expand them into metaphors and similes. Don't stick to nature and ideas you always hear in yoga classes. Play with ideas that speak to you, that create an image in your mind and a feeling in your body. This is your chance to put more of your personality into your teaching. It is also a great place to know your audience. If you are teaching a sports team, you can reference that sport, or anything specific to the people in the room that will help them relate to what you are saying.

Example: Lengthen

Lengthen up as if you are a rocket lifting off the earth.

Lengthen up like a child reaching for a chocolate.

AUTHORITY AND ESSENCE

When we are the teacher, we are the leader of the group. Being a leader means stepping into the role of authority. This doesn't have to be done with an attitude of higher status. In fact, it can be done gracefully with a welcoming attitude. Being the authority might be a challenge for your personality. Many of us have imposter's syndrome or some form of self-doubt that manifests as shyness or timidity in front of the group. If every teacher waited until they knew everything before teaching, we would have no teachers in the world. There is always more to learn; there is always the value of experience to lead you toward greater skill and knowledge. When we embrace the fact that we are where we are, we have enough knowledge to start. Then we must start. As you begin teaching or begin to incorporate new information and styles into your repertoire you might need to go back to Chapter 1 and revisit some of the work that empowers you and inspires confidence. It is interesting to monitor your feelings and reactions to the size of the group. If you identify as an introvert you might be more likely to react to a large or new group by retreating in some way. If you are more of an extrovert a larger group might give you a sense of strength. Again, knowing and relating to your unique experience will help you navigate and teach as a way of increasing self-awareness for your benefit. The more you accept the natural instincts you have the more you will be able to share your true self, which will resonate with students more than anything else.

You can use your language to help you find a sense of authority. Group instruction is by nature a direction, not an overly polite request or always a complete sentence. I often see female teachers struggle more with giving clear instructions. Look at the difference in the following:

Please perhaps place your hand under your shoulder.

Place your hand under your shoulder.

There is no need to use the voice of a drill sergeant, but the words themselves should be pared back to the essential and spoken without apology. Another word crutch I hear a lot of from yoga teachers (again, more common in my experience for female-identified teachers) is SORRY. It might be part of your cultural upbringing, so working on removing this word from your sentences unless you genuinely want to apologize is vital to speaking with confidence. I hear it in yoga instruction when it's not necessary and I hear it a lot in workshops or trainings as a precursor to a question or statement. We do not need to apologize for asking questions, for giving instructions, for sharing opinions or speaking our minds. Stop apologizing for taking up space. Try this exercise to practice getting your words clearer and more precise—with a friend preferably, but it is also possible with your recording device. This is a good one to do at lunch! You can listen to your recording and make your lunch following your own instructions.

Instruct someone on how to make your favorite sandwich. Be precise—how much of each ingredient, the order in which to place the fillings...

Now do it again with fewer words. In particular use fewer filler words and keep using the words that are clearest.

And again, even fewer words!

GOING INWARD: FINDING POWER

How does it feel to tell people what to do?

_____

_____

_____

_____

_____

Do you have a memory of a time you felt in charge of a group people? It might have been with family, children, work or any type of situation.

_____

_____

_____

_____

_____

Describe the inner and outer circumstances that led you to feel in charge.

_____

_____

_____

_____

Was this a positive experience?

_____

_____

_____

_____

_____

If not, what could have been different for it to be more positive?

_____

_____

_____

_____

_____

Describe your ideal teaching situation in detail. What are the circumstances that contribute to your feeling comfortable as the person in charge of the yoga room? Get really clear on this idea!

_____

_____

_____

_____

_____

_____

_____

_____

_____

_____

Pro tip

When you are teaching longer hours and developing your own content, take some time to set an intention for your career. One of my colleagues realized her ideal class is 12 people, some teachers want to focus on individual sessions, and others want to work primarily as trainers. There is no one path for a yoga teacher, and as you develop your career take time to make a business plan and set goals to help you chart the way that will be most fulfilling to you.

IMPROVISATION AND BODY LANGUAGE

ACTING ON THE MOMENT

Improvisation is a state of mind. It is an attitude of playfulness and flexibility, a way of seeing the world as full of possibilities instead of obstacles. The time I have spent playing improvisation games for theater has been monumental in helping my worldview open up toward positivity and humor. Improvisation is the total embodiment of moksha. In the last chapter we focused on physical techniques to create relaxation, release and freedom for our voices to gain emotional color as well as texture and power. Just as freedom is the underlying principle in voice work, it is also the key to improvisation.

In yogic philosophy we have the concept of the inner teacher. I like to picture my inner teacher as a Buddha-like angel, an older woman who is wise and content. In psychology and artistic process there is the concept of the inner critic. I often picture my inner critic as my high school acting teacher, Ms. G. She had a way of lifting one eyebrow that spoke volumes of disapproval. This one expression is burned into my memory and contributed through the years to many moments of self-censorship. In my mind the inner teacher and the inner critic are like the angel and devil archetypes that are often portrayed as sitting on each of our shoulders. In this binary vision there is a simplicity that can help us break free of the inner critic when that is the primary voice that holds us back from acting on our impulses and creative instincts. In a sense the inner teacher symbolizes our intuition, which when trusted always leads to a more interesting choice. As we expand ourselves on the path of yoga and life we are less caught in the illusion of a binary view of the world, and the non-duality of consciousness is more tangible.

Keith Johnstone writes about the creative process in *Impro: Improvisation and the Theatre*:

> My brain creates a whole universe without my having the least sense of effort... It's only when I believe my perceptions to be in error that I have to "do" anything. It's the same with imagination. Imagination is as effortless as perception, unless we think it might be "wrong," which is what our education encourages us to believe. Then we experience ourselves as "imagining," as "thinking up an idea," but what we're really doing is faking up the sort of imagination we think we ought to have.[11]

It is important to return again to the parallel concepts in yoga and art concerning process over product. In the research and development stages of any creative endeavor there must be freedom from editing. This moksha from the inner critic will not always be easy to find; it can be elusive and is always connected to our personal growth. I believe there is value in taking time to explore and aim to eradicate the inner critic for your expressive journey. Leave plenty of time for this section and if you need to take a break and come back to it, please don't give yourself a hard time. It's a great idea to build in time for self-care after you finish this bit. One of my theater teachers used to say that after a production he needed a hot chocolate to soothe his inner man. This might be a hot chocolate moment.

GOING INWARD: NAMING YOUR INNER CRITIC

Think back to a time that you tried, or wanted to try, something new. It can be simple like trying out a new hobby or weighty like trying out a new job, address or relationship. Write down what you wanted to try, and why.

_____

_____

_____

_____

Did you have doubts or second thoughts? If not, go back to the previous step and find something a little less simple, something that was not an easy thing to do.

_____

_____

_____

_____

What was the tone of voice inside your head during the doubts and second thoughts?

_____

_____

_____

_____

Do you recognize the voice? Does it remind you of anyone in your life?

_____

_____

_____

_____

If there is a person that embodies your "inner critic," name them now. Feel free to have more than one!

_____

_____

_____

_____

Send them gratitude for helping shape who you are right now. Write down your personal note of thanks here for safe keeping.

_____

_____

_____

_____

_____

_____

_____

_____

Acknowledge that you no longer need this voice if it is holding you back. When you hear it in the future you can name it, you can acknowledge that this voice is fear-based, that it is trying to keep you safe. Sometimes you can let it go. Sometimes not. It's part of your process.

_____

_____

_____

_____

Do something really nice for yourself now.

YES, AND

Improvisational theater has a rule that is not to be broken under any circumstances: Yes, And. This is an attitude that has helped me immensely to teach in a way that is authentic. The principle is simple: whatever is happening must be accepted before we add to it. Whether improvising a scene with someone or rehearsing from a script, this attitude gives actors the permission and responsibility to act in the moment. At a recent workshop a longtime yoga and meditation teacher commented that improvisation is very much like mindfulness. I totally agree. Mindfulness as a practice of being aware of what is present, what is actually happening versus being stuck in our thoughts and expectations, is the basis of improvisation.

Using this philosophy in daily life is an exercise in positivity. It is a great tool for looking at any situation from another angle: what can I add to this in a way that improves the world? As a yoga teacher it often will manifest as something along the lines of planning a class of backbends and then receiving a class with students dealing with spinal injuries. Being able to accept that the planned sequence needs to be modified or changed completely is the Yes. Another part of the Yes is acknowledging that you made an effort to plan the other sequence, and to acknowledge any emotional reaction you have to needing to change your plan, which might lead to another emotional reaction, and so on. Getting familiar with being honest with yourself, saying yes acceptingly to your own feelings, is step one in being present to find the And. The And is what you do with the situation you are in. What you add to the scene to drive the action forward. The And is how you react.

Being good at improvisation is just like anything else, you can get better the more you do it. Many people are terrified of playing theater games that involve improv. I meet people in my workshops who find this the most difficult ask, doing something without a plan. Being in the unknown is essentially a part of life. None of us really knows what is going to happen next. I find comfort in remembering that this is true for everyone.

PLAYING GAMES

Most improv games use more than one person. For this book I will include some individual improv exercises that you can do on your own to start building your improv muscles.

Pro tip
This is an attitude check. As you get to the level of teaching where you are teaching your curriculum multiple times to different groups, it can become easy to get stuck in a rut. Adopting an attitude of improvisation keeps it fresh, the way an actor needs to keep it fresh when playing the same part over and over. Allowing for play and seeing each student as a co-creator in the room will help rejuvenate any material.

Dancing with yourself

The lovely phrase "Dance like no one is watching" is a good tool for loosening up and getting out of your own way. Get some music that inspires you and boogie down on your own. The next step is to find some music that is not your typical dance music taste and improvise some dance steps to this music. Set a timer so that you are forced to continue even when it's challenging.

Present opening

Pantomime opening a box and take out the imaginary object. Use the object. Set a timer so you are forced to open a new box every 20 seconds. After a few rounds you might set the timer for shorter intervals so that you have to speed up. Speed is your friend in this game; it stops the inner critic from taking over and editing or planning what the next object will be. Avoid trying to be brilliant, just do the very first thing that comes to mind. This will help you to get more in touch with your impulses and out of your own box!

Gesture repetition

Gestures help articulate what you are saying; they are more than simply arm movements. Most gestures use the hands to demonstrate what you are saying. Choose a gesture that you feel comfortable doing. If you can't think of one that you often use or see, look ahead in this chapter at the list of body language and gestures (see "Body language clues" later in this chapter). Choose a common word, a linking word perhaps. One example to try is the word "and." Watch or listen to something (TV, news, podcast) for at least three minutes and each time you hear the word repeat your gesture. This will scramble the brain and start to get you accustomed to expressing more with your gestures. After you have done this game enough to feel clear with a few gestures, try the next level.

Next level gesture repetition is to memorize a short piece of text. It can be related to yoga or not, your choice. Aim for one minute or two. Set a timer to go off at random, surprise intervals. Use a gesture whenever the timer goes off. After this the next level is to use the same text and start to make your gestures big, wild, playful, even crazy. Maybe you can find gestures that use the whole body. It will become a bit like a mad dance, all done with the text so that you are speaking clearly and loudly. It should be fun and tiring. If there isn't some sweat on your upper lip, you aren't giving it enough enthusiasm.

Dialogue play

Turn on a show with the sound completely off. Improvise the dialogue of the characters. Use as many varied voices as you can. Warm your voice up first so that it is all done with an open throat and released jaw and face. Are you having fun yet?

Word association

Look around the room and choose one thing. Start a monologue on that object and without any pause delve into a long speech about it. Aim to include some personal experience—what does that object remind you of? No internal edit or filter here. Simply say the first things that come to mind.

Improv games in the yoga world

The following game is an adaptation of an exercise that Mick Napier calls Object Monologue.[12]

Write down ten of your favorite yoga asana and ten of your least favorite on small pieces of paper. Put them into a hat or bowl. Close your eyes. Pick one and do an instant workshop on that pose. Do not pause; go with your first idea. Challenge yourself to explain the pose without actually doing it. Use a timer to up the stakes. Extend the time so that you have to speak longer than usual about the pose. Then shorten it so you have to essentialize what you want to say about the pose.

After you have played this game you can uplevel. Add 20 themes that you might want to teach within the context of yoga. Write them on a different color of paper or put them in a different hat or bowl. Now choose a pose and a theme, with the same restrictions as the first level. Try different times, shorter or longer. Do not do the pose!

Body language is something you might not have thought about consciously; however, you are always using it in communication. What I find most compelling about body language as a theater artist and communication enthusiast is that it reveals more truth than people might want to show. It can be a window into the emotional reality so often obscured by social conditioning, just like the voice. One dictionary defines body language as "nonverbal, usually unconscious, communication through the use of postures, gestures, facial expressions, and the like."[13] If the yoga practice is meant to help us become more conscious, to shift us upward toward higher levels of consciousness, then without a doubt our body language is part of that journey.

Let's begin with the word "postures" from the above definition. In yoga asana practice we are literally using postures to shift our consciousness. We can use these postures to improve our overall health and strengthen our bodily systems, as well as using them to shift moods, the flow of energy, our perspective and our sense of connection. We need to bring what we learn on the yoga mat from the postures into our daily lives and our teaching lives. The reality for most of us is that we spend more time off the yoga mat than on it, so our posture and the impact it has on our body and mood when we are doing all the things we do (not just yoga!) are vital to our health and our ability to communicate effectively.

GOING INWARD: POSTURE CHECK

This is a tool I use throughout my day. I usually catch myself hunching over or crossing my legs habitually and twisting my spine in a less than helpful way. If working on a computer for extended amounts of time (more than an hour), try setting an alarm or using a reminder sticker note so that you check in every 20 minutes or so and release tension.

Mindfully, with soft eyes, see yourself as you actually are.

Notice right now how your posture is, what percentage of you is resting or leaning on something? What amount of muscular engagement is holding you up from gravity? Are you able to take a deep breath? Is there a habitual way of sitting or standing you are using now? What deeper patterns does this create in your fascia, your muscles and bones? Is your instinct to change immediately now that you are more conscious? Is the change creating an opposite effect, perhaps putting your body into another pattern of tension or overuse? What is a more balanced way of creating an efficient posture that feels sustainable? Start with small changes.

Take some notes here to reflect on what you found and the process.

_____

_____

_____

_____

_____

_____

_____

_____

Our bodies are an expression of each experience we have lived. Body language is one of the patterns that create our posture. An ideal yoga practice will improve posture, gradually through dedication and consistency. We must begin by noticing our habits and working slowly enough to allow the process to unfold at a rate that we can maintain and integrate with daily life. One of my teachers in graduate school remarked that she had done years of theater training through Alexander and Feldenkrais techniques, yet offstage or out of the training room she felt her posture was horrible. This is one of the takeaways I hope to give you—your daily posture is perhaps more important to your overall health than your "practice." Postural awareness is a skill, not meant to keep you hyperfocused on yourself or any idea of perfection. It is a skill that ideally gives you the physical openness to express freely whatever you are feeling and want to communicate. If we close ourselves off with the common position of rounded shoulders and closed chest, we show the world we are protecting ourselves, trying to hide and be literally closed off to others. When we stand with one hip hiked upward, bearing weight asymmetrically through the legs it sends a message that we are unstable, and when we cross our arms it says we are rejecting, denying or blocking. These are general interpretations and there are many models that exist for classifying body language. To learn for yourself simply take an outing to people watch. Watch from afar so you cannot hear any words. Notice how when you watch people a lot is revealed about their inner state.

To see body language in its purest form, try the following exercise. It's one of my favorites from my theater training and I use it regularly with students in my workshops and trainings.

Stocking mask

This is best done with a friend or colleague. It offers a lot of giggling at the beginning, which is great for your diaphragm. If you don't have anyone to play with, use a full-length mirror, preferably at a bit of distance to give you enough space to see your whole body.

Take an opaque stocking of a very dark color and cut it halfway.

Stand in front of the mirror or friend and try different positions to see how, without any facial expression getting in the way, you can clearly see a whole story just in the way you stand.

Below are some playful examples of body postures I often observe in teachers. Take a look and notice what your instinctive reaction is. Does it pull you in or push you away? Does it inspire a story in your mind?

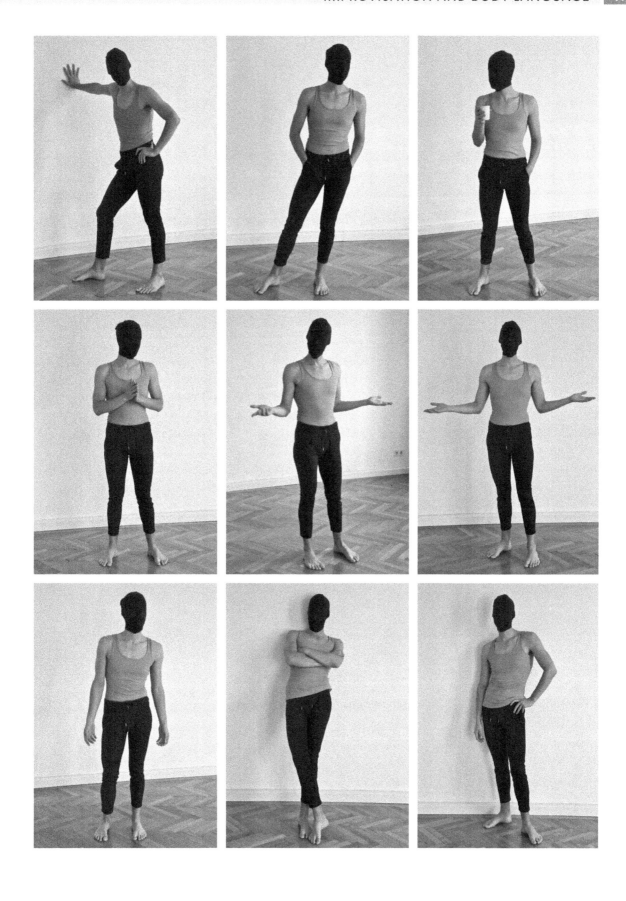

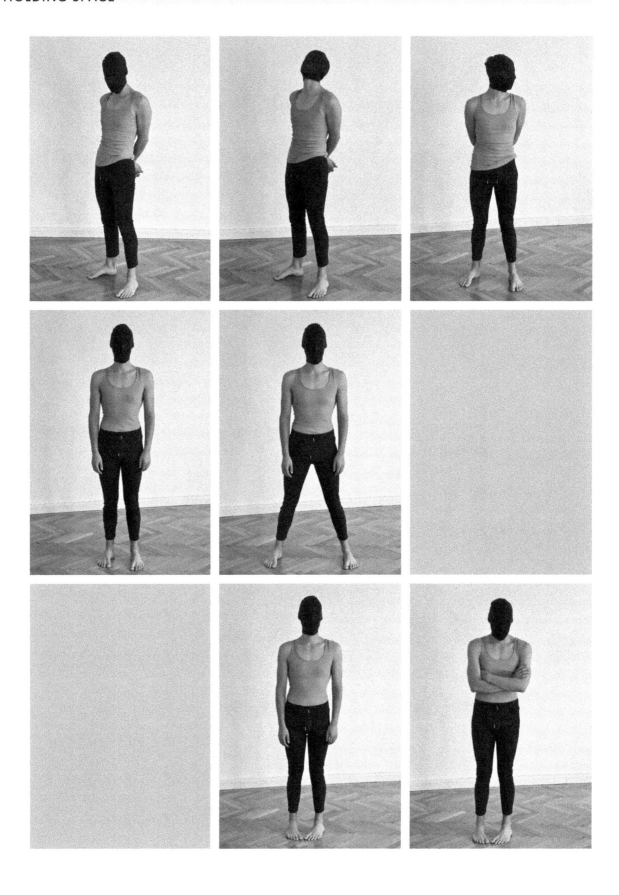

Body language clues

Here are some common theories on patterns of body language and gesture that can help you as you begin to look at yourself and others. Many of them are in the context of conversation, but elements can be applied to teaching when you begin to notice your tendencies.

Closing is a pattern of defending, hiding, refusing and denying:

- crossing arms or legs, pulling in shoulders, elbows and knees to protect organs and vulnerable parts

- turning hands from palms up to palms down

- curling fingers into the palm, protecting them (and also making a fist)

- turning feet to point toes inwards

- hunching down, with any or all of the above, making the body less threatening and a smaller target.

Crossing is a pattern associated with protecting, similar to *closing*:

- crossing arms across the body

- crossing just the hands or wrists

- holding hands

- intertwining the fingers

- crossing legs, either above the knee or at the ankles.

Enacting or *shaping* is a complex pattern of acting out thoughts:

- gesticulating with hands to show an idea, such as pounding a fist in anger

- re-enacting or acting out an idea

- pantomime

- arms and hands make shapes to reinforce words.

Moving away (not only a change of space between people) often shows refusal or denial:

- pulling back the head in fear, confusion or surprise

- pulling back arms or shoulders

- hollowing the chest, pulling it back

- turning away the head and, in the extreme, showing the back.

Moving forward is usually seeking or even attacking:

- reaching forward with arms and hands, giving, grabbing or striking
- pushing the head forward
- pressing hips forward
- leaning forward
- stepping forward.

Opening is a pattern of readiness to listen, acceptance and vulnerability or trust:

- raising the head from a chin-down position to looking forward
- unfolding arms
- holding open palms
- spreading palms in an opening circular move around from front to side
- turning hands over from palms-down to palms-up
- pointing toes outwards, with splayed feet
- standing with legs wide.

Preening is either insecurity, comfort seeking or flirtation:

- touching arms or hands or other part of the body in self-comfort
- cleaning hair, face or clothing
- stroking arms or hugging oneself.

Repetition often shows boredom, impatience, irritation, tension or repressed impulses:

- nodding or shaking the head
- tapping the teeth
- waggling the eyebrows
- swinging the arms
- clapping of hands
- waving with hands
- drumming of fingers
- swinging or bouncing a leg
- tapping of feet.

Striking usually shows aggression or enthusiasm—the body can be used in various ways to symbolically strike out at others:

- wagging a finger in admonishment

- shaking an entire arm

- jabbing a finger toward someone, as if prodding them

- poking a finger into an open hand or onto a table

- slapping a fist into an open hand or onto a table

- stamping the ground with a foot.

THE RULE(S) OF PERSONAL COMMUNICATION

Prof. Albert Mehrabian conducted famous studies in the 1970s at the University of California at Los Angeles (UCLA) looking at efficacy in communication He concluded with what is referred to as the Mehrabian Rule of Personal Communication or the 7-38-55 rule. The findings postulate that only 7 percent of what people understand comes from our words, while 38 percent is from tone of voice and 55 percent from body language and facial gesture.

When I first came across this I was really surprised. I was raised to believe that what I said was more important than how I said it. Does research prove otherwise? Not necessarily, as the Mehrabian Rule is way too simple. Later studies and criticisms of Mehrabian's conclusions highlight the difficulties involved in studying communication, and he himself cautioned that his study focused on conveying feelings and attitudes rather than information.

There are many models of communication, and none that is foolproof. As you can see from the above list, gestures and body language are often interpreted differently. We can only generalize to a certain degree.

Regardless of all these factors, I still think this a wonderful reminder about how important body language, gesture, facial expression, vocal tone and inflection truly are. When we do not align our words with these elements then we lose our authenticity, which is one of the most important elements in yoga teaching.

This information made me re-evaluate a lot of my communication, not just my teaching. This affirms my belief in the importance of following our "gut instincts" and trusting our intuition. The emotional state of others is something we feel and understand; we get the meaning of what someone says even if the words are not necessarily clear. I encounter this on a daily basis now that I live in a country where I am not fluent in the language. It is amazing how much I can understand even if I have no idea what exactly they are saying. Current neuroscientific research on mirror neurons confirms this phenomenon. Mirror neurons are responsible for learning, language, empathy and imitation—basically all that makes us social animals. Marco Iacoboni, a neuroscientist at the University of California at Los Angeles, explains how mirror neurons function:

> The way mirror neurons likely let us understand others is by providing some kind of inner imitation of the actions of other people, which in turn leads us to "simulate" the intentions and emotions associated with those actions. When I see you smiling, my mirror neurons for smiling fire up, too, initiating a cascade of neural activity that evokes the feeling we typically associate with a smile. I don't need to make any inference on what you are feeling, I experience immediately and effortlessly (in a milder form, of course) what you are experiencing.[14]

This idea, that when we are in dialogue with someone our neurons are actually mirroring the neurons of the speaker, could be seen as an evolutionary function to give humans empathy. I know this as something that can be felt, like when you have a conversation with someone that just "flows" or seems "effortless." This is more than just a feeling—it is actually happening on a chemical and physical level. Next time you are enjoying a conversation where you feel the connection deeply with your conversation partner or with a presenter or teacher, remember that your mirror neurons are at work.

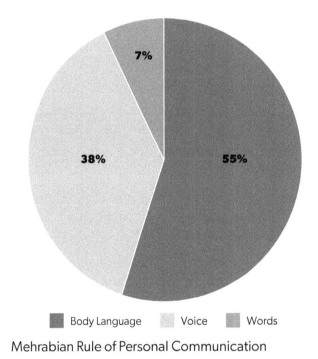

Mehrabian Rule of Personal Communication

The power of a smile: putting mirror neurons to the test

Smiling can be especially contagious—notice when you walk down the street and a smiling stranger catches your eye. Even at the grumpiest moment it is hard not to smile back. Now that we know why (mirror neurons) we can make an informed choice to smile as a way to potentially shift our own energy, relax our facial muscles as we release the smile and maybe shift the energy of a student, the class or a stranger. I'm not advocating a "grin and bear it" mentality or encouraging you to smile in a fake way that would cover up an honest emotion. I am pointing out that being aware of our own energy and knowing that it has an effect on those around us is important. Students are attracted to different teachers because they get something from the teaching, and energetic exchange takes place when we teach. We can see this as simply mirror neurons at work, we can see it as the sequencing or style of yoga being taught, and we can acknowledge that our subtle and emotional bodies are also a huge part of any exchange.

The next factor that influences the way people understand us is vocal quality. This is not simply whether we have a pleasing voice, which is of course highly subjective, but has more to do with the emotional tone of the voice matching up with what we are saying. The voice reveals our inner state, and this is what people are reacting to. Regardless of technical training, we must find an authenticity that allows our speech to be aligned with our meaning. Another aspect of this factor is the way our voice matches what we are doing. If there is a disconnect between what we are thinking and feeling and the words we are using, it is clear that the audience or listener will know this, no matter what words we choose. Again, naming what you actually feel and acknowledging it to yourself has the power to break through any masks that might be blocking your ability to connect. Being able to honestly acknowledge your interior will have an immense impact on your ability to be present with the exterior, or the people you are with and the place you are in.

When you feel yourself repressing your inner state, take a break of even one breath and acknowledge how you feel. In many professional situations (I consider yoga teaching a profession!) it would be inappropriate to say this out loud. However, there is a difference between ignoring and creating a barrier of falsity versus accepting what is and incorporating it in a way that allows you to be present to your task at hand. We will revisit this in Chapter 8.

5

STAGING

One of the most powerful tools I have learned from theater is to partner with whatever comes. It goes back to Chapter 4 on improvisation. This technique is mirrored in the Buddhist idea of accepting what is. It is echoed in the yogic philosophy of right knowledge, of being present to reality. Whatever role we find ourselves in, our ability to get out of our heads, out of the trappings of expectations and ego-driven storylines, and open ourselves to what is actually happening is the key—to doing a good "job" and being present. This chapter shifts the view and uses the lens of theater to explore how the yoga teaching experience can be enhanced for both teacher and students.

When I see the room, the people and all the circumstances of my environment as my partners and not obstacles they feed me inspiration. In the physical theater vocabulary of Mary Overlie and Anne Bogart, called "viewpoints," we are taught that the space and architecture of where we are is just as relevant and pregnant with potential as another actor or any other element in the play. The process of seeing the world like this can be a gradual learning, and I hope you will start to see the world with freshness as you test these concepts.

GOING INWARD: OBSERVING THE OUTER WORLD

Take a moment wherever you are and breathe deeply. Notice your feet. Your breath. Any tension in your body you can release, release it. Read these next words and then put the book down: look out and notice something you have never seen about the location you are in. Maybe a corner of the room, maybe the floor, the ceiling, the angles of the light. Find something interesting to you about the space and simply observe it.

Notice how that shifts your awareness. Does it change the tempo of thoughts or sharpness in the mind? Maybe it was a challenge to stop your inner chatter and simply see with your eyes.

Note down your experience.

_____

_____

_____

_____

_____

In a moment after you have read this, close your eyes and listen without any intention other than hearing the sounds around you. Do this for at least a minute, perhaps setting a timer to help you.

How did that go? How many thoughts do you have connected to the sounds around you? Did your mind find the ability to simply be present to the sounds?

_____

_____

_____

_____

_____

OBSERVATION ON YOUR FEET: WALKING IN THE SPACE

This is best done in a large room, or even outside where you have a lot of space to move freely. I like to do this exercise in public spaces where there are crowds to navigate. Airports and shopping malls are great for this! The object is to walk freely at a pace slightly faster than your casual walk, responding to the impulses of what you see and feel around you. Give yourself at least 20 minutes to play this game. Music is helpful if you are in a public place. Allow your headphones to give you permission to move differently from how you often do. With an efficient and quick walking pace your body will have a heightened sense of where you are. Continue to observe with your eyes as in the previous exercise, letting what you see pull you toward it or push you away. Notice how your gut can communicate with you, how intuition can guide you. You do not need an explanation or rationale for why you want to walk toward something or away, whether the buildings make you want to dance or flee; continue to let go of your thinking mind and tune in to your body. Let it guide you.

Make some notes on what you discover. The more you play with this exercise, the easier it will get to feel your instincts guiding you.

_____

_____

_____

_____

_____

NEXT LEVEL: WALKING IN THE SPACE AS A SOCIAL EXPERIMENT

The next step in this exercise is usually done in a group where everyone has the instructions. It is also a very revealing exercise to do in public on your own; however, it will take a little more *chutzpah* or guts to do this as a solo project. I encourage you to try it when you have played with the previous level at least a few times and are getting comfortable with these outer-focused meditations.

Go out into the world with an attitude of curiosity toward yourself. This requires a complete letting go of judgment. The point is to notice when your judgments arise (which they inevitably will!) and let them go (the hardest part). As you walk through the space (street, mall, airport) notice as well your instincts toward the environment and toward the people. Which people are you attracted to (not only in the sexual regard)? Which people are you averse to? When do you feel a genuine impulse to smile, or nod? When is the smile or nod simply a social construction, something you habitually do because you have been taught it is correct behavior? Are you able to drop those "inauthentic" smiles and reactions, in favor of something more honest and authentic? Can you look people in the eyes as you walk? Can you look someone in the eyes with a "neutral" expression? Simply look at them and notice your inner reactions, sensing more and more your own instincts. This exercise is a very challenging one for most of us. Our social conditioning is usually very strong and often so deep that we do not even feel the difference between a true instinct and a social habit.

I am not an advocate for dropping all social conventions in any circumstance. I do, however, think it is important that you get to know yourself and find out whether you are able to be authentic around others and in contact. On the street some people make contact, and some are totally immersed in their inner life. This exercise is about staying connected to your inner world and gradually making contact and feeling comfortable with both. Maybe start with this exercise. This is a wonderful way to start questioning our motives and why we react to certain people with attraction and others with aversion. Some people remind us (consciously or unconsciously) of someone from the past, and we carry so many experiences within us that it is vital when you work with people to accept that there are many factors involved within each of us that create the dynamics of relationship.

When I am teaching I want to be conscious of who I am drawn to and who I feel wary of, I want to question whether I am safely working within my personal boundaries and also maintaining a sense of fairness in terms of who gets my attention in the class. As people walk into class, how do I greet them? Does my face feel frozen in a polite mask, or can I actually allow a real reaction as I see each person and notice my inner state? These are the questions I ask myself continually. I believe that students are picking up on whether we are actually there for them or stuck in ourselves and trapped by our ideas of what a yoga teacher should be and how they should behave. I will explain more about how to bridge the gaps and deal with students in an authentic way that honors your true feelings and is also "polite" in Chapter 7.

What was fun for you to explore?

_____

_____

_____

What was challenging?

_____

_____

_____

Did you surprise yourself in any way?

_____

_____

_____

Would you try this again?

_____

_____

_____

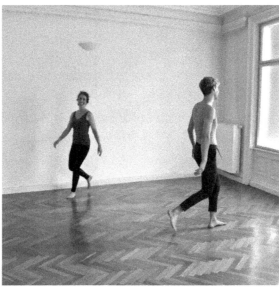

THE THREE CIRCLES OF ATTENTION

Konstantin Stanislavski (1863(?)–1938) was a Russian theater master whose work had a huge influence on theater internationally. His theory on how to create *naturalism*—acting that is as close to reality as possible—was revolutionary in his time. He identified what he coined "three circles of attention" that an actor must use. I think of them as levels of awareness. The first circle is understood as *solitude in public*. This is our awareness of ourselves. Some teachers lose their ability to focus on themselves, to the point of dehydration! Keeping your own body safe, knowing your limits and boundaries, is the first necessity in teaching. From there the second circle is the actor's concentration on the other characters in the play/other actors on stage. In yoga teaching this is our concentration on the students. This is where listening and responding to the group is so similar to acting, where we are listening and responding to our fellow actors. Next is the third circle, which for Stanislavski was the entire production—the crew, the set, the audience, the theater, etc. In yoga teaching this is our set, our props (literally!), the music, the light, the studio, the events of the day, the receptionist, the heating—everything about where we are.

THE GROUND

In yoga and meditation practice the ground of the practice is you: body, mind, spirit. In theater the ground is the stage. What type of stage you work on is really important. You have to be aware of the angle of a raked stage, your sight lines in a proscenium or a theater in the round. I find it similar in the yoga room. Some of my favorite rooms to teach in have difficult shapes, or columns in the middle that give a restricted view. I like these challenges, and being aware of the students *and* the space allows me to look for solutions that often complement or even create the theme of the class.

For example, when teaching outside, the grass and uneven ground is a fantastic point to highlight the foundation of each pose and how we connect with the earth. In a room with columns, using them to do poses at the wall is a great way to utilize the space and help people have the room they need to try inversions. Choosing how the mats are laid is really important to how you feel standing at the "front" of the room. Equally, knowing that you have space on the sides of the room if you need to demonstrate poses that use the mat in a horizontal orientation and making your way there without tripping on props or stepping on people might seem basic but does take a bit of forethought. Tripping over props and stepping on students is unfortunately really easy to do if we are not connected to the place and more likely to happen if we are focused too much on ourselves or where we are walking to instead of the actual journey.

Getting comfortable in the room is key to being present in teaching. This requires you to be aware of the environment and the details around you—the more details you are aware of, the more creative material you have and the more awake you will be as you teach. A lot of awkward moments can be avoided by taking the time to check out where you work, which is extremely relevant when you are in a new space. Recognizing these elements as part of your class will start to influence your ability to improvise and create a class that is relevant to the moment.

Thinking about the experience of your students, from when they walk in to when they leave, can help you choose where to teach and also give you a lot of information about the kind of students or audience that you work with. The studio with the lovely tea and the fresh fruit is a great example of an ambience that students are drawn to. One of my teachers, Uma Dinsmore-Tuli, taught in her pregnancy teacher training to use flowers and beautiful altar objects to help women feel inspired from the moment they walk into the room. In a gym the vibe will be different and finding the place that supports your style, that creates a great backdrop for your work is important. Think about where you like to practice yoga and seek out spaces that feel welcoming, where you walk in and take a deep breath. For practical reasons when you are a new teacher, traveling or working privately in some else's space you might not be able to be so choosy. However, you can be aware of what you are working with or in some cases what you might even feel you are working against. Knowing that this will affect your teaching and figuring out how to accept it and let it become a positive influence when possible is the main learning curve.

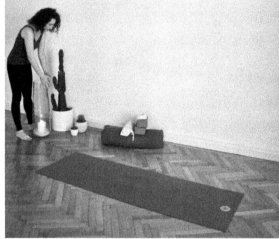

PROPS

I'm very clear with my students about where to put their props, especially as I like to use a lot of props. This is for my own safety as when I walk through the room to adjust and find my light, I need to be free from walking through an obstacle course of dangerous yoga bricks. Teachers and students have been seriously injured from tripping on props, so make sure you have a clear path to walk instead of a cluttered one! Some of my theater training in Viewpoints with the SITI Company in New York focused on how the pattern of our feet affects us. If you are snaking around the room and focusing on the floor, then your attention is not where it is most useful. You need to be able to look out and see your students, so taking an extra minute to tell people to keep props neat and not leave their stuff on the floor is worth it. Your voice is not going to be well projected if you are looking at the floor either.

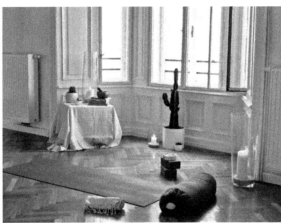

COSTUME

Another seemingly obvious point: you have got to be comfortable in your clothes. If you can't practice without having to tug your trousers up or your shirt down, then you definitely can't teach in them. I see a lot of teachers wearing clothes that look great until they start moving around, and if you are tugging at your clothing it does not help you to project confidence. Give your teaching clothes a test run and check that they aren't see-through or showing off your undies. I've seen more yoga teachers' undies than I care to remember—please keep it decent. It will make you and your students more comfortable, which is a huge step toward teaching authentically and feeling your power as a speaker.

DISRUPTIONS

I have taught countless classes in rooms where outside noise from the street or other rooms in the building pull focus and can create a sense of distraction or aggravation. Using these outer sounds as inspiration to create a theme of listening without judgment and using mindfulness instructions to help people embrace the moment as part of their practice have led to some very powerful sessions. Sometimes it is as simple as naming it once. Acknowledging that there is something going on rather than ignoring it can break the ice and help everyone realize they are not alone in their feelings.

Interruptions

People coming in late or trying to come in late are one kind of interruption that is really common. I'll talk about my ideas on holding boundaries for this in Chapter 7. Following the rule of improvisation will help you deal with the following common interruptions:

- power fail

- music fail

- yoga props broken, missing or not enough for the group

- people entering late

- people leaving early

- fire alarm

- extremely loud sirens outside

- phone ringing

- pregnant woman showing up in non-pregnancy class

- pregnant woman going into labor (true story!)

- talkative students.

GOING INWARD: INTERRUPTIONS

Think about how you would handle the situations above. As quickly as possible, what are your first ideas? Then pause and consider what is going to support the type of ambience you are aiming for with your classes.

_____

_____

_____

_____

_____

Now list some other possible surprises and how you might handle them gracefully.

_____

_____

_____

_____

_____

Outside noise

This is one of the biggest issues for yoga teachers everywhere. Inevitably, outside noise will at some point play a role in your work. The world is noisy. It's vital that you know and find ways to deal with outside sound distractions. For example, if there is construction outside, what could you adjust in your sequence to accommodate keeping the windows closed on a hot day? Taking it a step further, how can you acknowledge that noise without giving it the power to completely derail your class? One of my favorite ways of doing this is to create a theme on listening inward. When I introduce the theme I suggest that the noise outside is something we can work with to strengthen our practice. I often use outside sounds for a listening meditation. Another layer to this is having the intention to notice our reactions to noise mindfully, to see it symbolically as the noise in our heads. The most interesting themes can come from your ability to notice what is happening in the environment of your class and use it almost like another character to play with. It takes you out of the annoyance that is a common reaction to anything "disturbing," like unexpected loud construction, and puts you in the position to play and interact with awareness. It gives you a levity that embodies being open to the moment. This approach also helps you keep the teaching fresh, as of course each class will have something different happening that you can choose to explore.

Pro tip
Talking over other students, raising your voice to grab attention when the partner exercise needs to be finished or calling out "Listen up!" are some of the easiest ways to strain your voice. In trainings and workshops, when we give the students group and partner work, using a bell or even a clap is the safest way to get the room back without hurting your voice. I usually explain the need for silence as soon as the bell rings when I start the day or training as one of the ground rules. When the siren screams and the noise level jumps, take the moment to be silent until the loudness stops. Fighting against these noises is not worth the effort or risk to your voice.

MUSIC: TO PLAY OR NOT TO PLAY

Yet another hot debate topic in the yoga world is about the role of music in classes. Some studios and teachers are known for their playlists more than the actual teaching or style of yoga. Other teachers never use music, or only use music that is instrumental. I have enjoyed Vinyasa Flow classes with hip hop and pop music. I have hated music in other classes. Music is personal. Everyone will have a different reaction. I encourage you to find your happy medium with music. Do not rely on it to create the entire mood for you. Let the music support your sequence, and support your voice, not upstage it. It's a sad moment for me when the music is louder than the teacher. If your voice is challenged, recognize that the music is another hurdle for you to get your voice over. I recommend being able to teach without it so that if the music fails, it doesn't ruin the class!

FIND YOUR MARK AND CHEAT OUT

Light is important, and in evening classes some teachers keep the lights low to invite students toward relaxation. This is fantastic for creating mood as long as your students can see you when you need them to! It is also worth noting that students who have experienced trauma or are unfamiliar with yoga might have a very difficult experience in a low lit room and feel unsafe. Some locations have shadowy lights and you will need to "find your light" as we say in the theater. I think of this as my technique for sight lines also, and I look at the room in terms of finding where the most people can see me best. In theater we call this cheating out or staying open to the audience. It might be more natural to turn to someone when speaking, but if that puts my back to the rest of the group then I will stand at an angle so that I am still open to the majority of the students. This is a worthwhile challenge when adjusting students. Being open to the audience means that my voice will be better projected, that I will be visible and that I am able to see my students. Staying open is always on my mind when I teach a group. During the class this means I need to be aware of how the sequence changes the direction people are facing, so that if the class is twisting toward the right and I want to show a new pose, I make sure I am on the right side of the room ready to demonstrate before they arrive. When people are in a balancing pose, I am careful not to walk across their line of vision, which would disturb their balance. I want my place in the room, and whether I am still or moving (adjusting, mirroring, etc.), to shore up the teaching, not undermine it. Just as your journey as a yoga practitioner is characterized by moments when you become more awakened to something in your life, this is a way of awakening to the art of teaching. Day by day you will start to see the rooms you work in with new eyes.

GOING INWARD: SENSIBILITY TO SPACE

Start by asking yourself these questions to start increasing your sensibility to space:

Where is my favorite place to teach?

_____

_____

_____

_____

_____

Where is my favorite place to practice?

_____

_____

_____

_____

_____

What shape is the room? Is it round, narrow, does it have any special features? Are the ceilings high or low?

_____

_____

_____

_____

_____

What are the smells, sounds, textures?

_____

_____

_____

_____

_____

What are the acoustics like?

_____

_____

_____

_____

Where are the lights, fan, stereo hook-ups, etc.?

_____

_____

_____

_____

Do I feel connected to the space? Why?

_____

_____

_____

_____

Are there rituals I enjoy in setting up the space (lighting candles, opening windows, organizing props, etc.)?

_____

_____

_____

_____

How can I create an environment that is welcoming? What is needed for the students to have a fuller experience?

_____

_____

_____

_____

_____

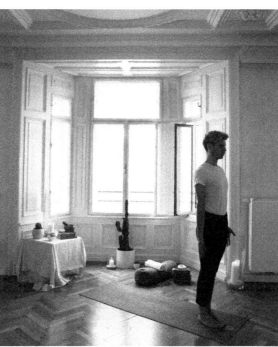

All of this is a way for you to take the stage or take your place as the teacher and embrace the spotlight so that your teaching can shine. If it triggers an emotional reaction, you are not alone! Being looked at is not something most of us embrace, as it can easily feel like we are being judged and not just seen. Take some time now to practice being seen. Allowing yourself to be seen in your full humanity will give your students permission to be themselves.

Go to a mirror. Look yourself in the eyes. Let go of criticism, let go of noticing parts of yourself you would change. Let go of appreciating your favorite parts. Simply see.

Reflections on your reflection:

_____

_____

_____

_____

_____

_____

_____

_____

_____

6

HOW WE LEARN

As teachers we can easily forget how it felt when yoga was new and not as easy for us. This chapter is a window into the process of learning. Even though you have been learning your whole life, you might not have actually studied how it happens. There are many philosophies and ideas on how we learn, most of which are based on research for academic institutions. I find it disheartening that most training programs for yoga teachers have little to no information on how humans learn. I consider the profession of yoga teaching as part of the field of education, so for me it is important to be aware of how my students learn. This helps me support their process with more than clever sequences. I have taken some simple techniques that are used by professional teachers and applied them to the physical process of learning asana. We will start this chapter with some reminders about the nervous system and motor cortex to refresh your memory on how the brain learns movement.

THE SCIENCE OF LEARNING

The central nervous system is made up of the cerebrum, cerebellum, brainstem and spinal cord. The brainstem is in charge of automatic activities like heartbeat, breathing and swallowing. The cerebellum helps muscles work together for coordination, balance and learned movements. The cerebrum is where learning, thinking, remembering, emotions, feeling sensations and voluntary muscle movement take place. The motor cortex is a special part of the cerebrum that sends signals to the rest of the body in order to move. It signals muscle groups to relax or engage, via the spinal cord.

The nervous system and muscles act together to achieve movement of or within the body. Signals that trigger movement are generated in the brain or spinal cord and then travel along motor neurons to the muscles. The signals travel very rapidly along the nerve cells and are transmitted chemically or electrically from one neuron to another across tiny gaps called synapses. Signals also are sent along sensory neurons from muscles and sensing organs to the spinal cord or brain.[15]

An adult who no longer uses the cerebrum to learn new movements on a regular basis will need to create new pathways in the brain when they begin to practice yoga. This can be a huge challenge, especially when we consider that when pathways in the brain are not being used they are regularly sent less energy and the pathways disintegrate. For those of us who teach beginners, or if you are teaching a new pose or a very different way of breathing or moving, we need to remember what is happening for our students on a neurological level. It may not be that students lack the mobility or the strength for certain poses; it could simply be that they are so different to their habitual movements that the cerebrum hasn't had a chance to make the connection.

The good news is that current research into how these pathways are created, maintained or lost has proven that new pathways can be created, and old pathways unearthed. This process of forming or rebuilding pathways is called neuroplasticity. The fact that at any age our brains are capable of growing new neurons and creating new wiring for new information was a huge discovery for the science and educational communities. Previously, it was thought that at maturity the brain would no longer be able to create new wiring systems. It is clear that with age this process slows down, but the brain is so dynamic that it actually never stops rewiring and repurposing.

When the body is able to perform a new physical or motor task, it takes a lot of practice until that way of moving is actually learned. What I mean by "learned" is that at some point, which is different for each individual, the pathway that the neuron signals travel as you perform a motor task will change. As you get better at the task it will shift and the pathway will no longer be from the cerebrum to the motor cortex; it will instead be a message coming from the cerebellum. It is as if the cerebellum learns the new task from the understanding of the cerebrum, but only when you have repeated it enough! This reinforces the idea of yoga as a practice—practice is the embodiment of learning.

GOING INWARD: MOTOR LEARNING RECALL

Think of something that was physically challenging for you to learn as a child. Maybe it was riding a bicycle, roller skating or using chopsticks. Can you recall how long it took until you were able to do this action? How long until you could do it well? Were there moments along the learning process that were frustrating? Exhilarating? Take a few moments and write some of your memories and how it felt to go through the learning process. Notice what emotions come to mind in relation to these memories.

_____

_____

_____

_____

_____

The process

Memory is a key component in learning. Our working memory is what both gathers new information and uses it. This memory has low capacity and is easily overwhelmed. This is the same part of our memory that controls our behavior moment to moment. Knowing that the trend toward multitasking, multi-screens and the constant stream of distraction from our devices is making an impact on our capacity to concentrate gives me a clear guideline when I plan classes and workshops. Too much information is referred to as *cognitive overload*. When I first started leading all-day workshops and teacher trainings I was so eager to deliver as much content as possible that I often didn't give enough breaks. Students were overwhelmed. Taking a break every couple of hours is not just important for taking care of the body; the mind also needs a break. In order to actually integrate the information I am teaching I now build in more short breaks whenever possible. I also avoid lecturing without using games, teaching devices and creative techniques to keep the focus. I aim my lectures at no more than one hour without an interactive or experiential element.

It is becoming widely accepted that more than just our cognitive capacity, or IQ, controls how we learn. Our emotional state has a huge effect on our ability to learn. Situations where students feel stressed, shamed or just uncomfortable make it more difficult for them to learn. This is really important when considering teaching yoga within different cultural contexts. Yoga studios have a culture of their own, especially here in the Western world. Many people are not accustomed to taking off their shoes, let alone their socks, in a public space. It might seem completely normal to you and totally foreign to one of your students. Being sensitive and aware, not only of the differences in culture from one country or ethnic group to another but also of the culture of yoga in the environment in which you are holding your classes or meeting your students, will help you ease your students into being comfortable enough to learn. This is one of the skills that truly sets great teachers apart. I have been in classes where teachers shamed people for being late, yelled at people for not following along or demanded that socks be taken off. This type of authoritarian teaching might appeal to some people, but it does not help the learning process. This ties in to how you set the stage for your class, whether you are speaking with respect and nonviolent communication techniques and how you level the field for all students to feel welcome.

Another necessary part of learning is making mistakes. As difficult as it is for most of us to imagine failure, it is a big part of the process. The key is to focus on starting again. Shifting our attention away from the mistake is easier if we have an attitude of accepting that making mistakes is a natural element when learning new skills. When we draw too much attention to the mistake we reinforce "incorrect" pathways in the brain and make it more difficult for "correct" pathways to be fully formed. Letting go of the mistake is the key for making the new neural pathway.

GOING INWARD: FREEDOM TO FAIL

If you're anything like me, making mistakes was not encouraged during most of my educational career. Learning to allow mistakes is key for not only improvisation and creativity, but all learning. Take some time now to question your relationship to making mistakes.

Has anything shifted since you began looking at this topic in your life and in your teaching?

_____

_____

_____

_____

_____

How do you react when you perceive that you have made a mistake in your teaching?

_____

_____

_____

_____

_____

What types of circumstances make it easier for you to let go and move on from mistakes that happen when you are teaching?

_____

_____

_____

_____

_____

How is your reaction to mistakes during teaching similar or different to when you make mistakes in other areas of your life?

_____

_____

_____

_____

_____

Write about a moment when you made a mistake in a class or during teaching. How did you react in front of the student(s)? How did you feel? Did you let it go? Did you learn anything?

_____

_____

_____

_____

_____

_____

_____

_____

_____

_____

Our attitude toward failure and mistakes, whether we give an open space for the process of learning or whether we are product oriented, underlies the way that we teach. As a young teacher I had less tolerance for mistakes, more need for the asana to be perfected as opposed to explored. With time my approach has grown and evolved toward inquiry-based learning and teaching, so that I am encouraging my students to learn with me and share in the process rather than simply construct poses.

It turns out that our brains need novelty. Boredom has one of the most limiting effects on our ability to learn. The dopamine we get from a new situation can help the brain to focus and retain information, as well as provide an extra kick of motivation. Something as simple as having people put their mats in different spots or creating a sequence that shifts people's orientation to another part of the room can be the change that makes a difference for brains to wake up a little more.

In Chapter 7 I will talk about teaching techniques, which are often presented as ways to engage different learning styles. Some people are labeled as audio learners, visual learners, kinesthetic learners, etc. My initial research into this field, over ten years ago, led me to lots of information on these so-called types of learners. At the moment we are seeing more and more that everyone is some combination and that parceling out the learning styles is not that efficient in creating teaching methods. It turns out the emotional and social situation has more impact on a student than whether their preferred learning "style" is being catered to. This requires us as educators to look at how the "soft skills" of communication and underlying emotional states of students are affecting learning.

Keeping up with what you learn is key. Just as new pathways can be created, they can also be neglected and then the brain sends fewer nutrients and upkeep falls short. Continuing to engage with the material (whatever it is) is one of the only ways to truly retain information and skills in the long run. Most people need a social environment to learn best, which is good to remember for planning courses and classes. A safe, encouraging community environment is the best way to facilitate learning.

TRAINING MODELS

For those of us who lead teacher trainings or day-long immersion workshops, there are many formats to choose from. At the moment most yoga training is centered on either a 200-hour or 300-hour format. The teaching time is usually done as a residential or intensive type of training, sometimes with students in class up to ten hours per day, or weekends or modules spread out over a set period of time. I do think that some people prefer to learn in an intensive situation; they are perhaps supported by the tight-knit community feeling that often accompanies a residential intensive training. They might also want an exotic location as destination teacher trainings are more and more popular today. If you are planning trainings, it is important to think about what type of format will work best for the learners. Of course, cost, calendar and taking into account the students' work schedule will be part of the decision process. Building into any full day of training enough breaks and cumulative learning so that the material is repeated in a way that students will remember it is key. I notice in the yoga industry there is often a lot of information given in workshops or short training modules with the emphasis being on more information in a short amount of time. This is often to accommodate the financial reality of traveling teachers having high expenses and often high pay demands from local studios. The yoga industry doesn't exist in a vacuum, trainings and information are considered commodities and as such most consumers are trying to get more for their money. I believe that this underlying attitude has a detrimental effect on yoga teaching and the process of learning. I hope that the industry and the community of yoga teachers will help to shift our educational models toward learner-friendly and process-oriented models. As you are reading this book it is starting now with you.

Across all types of classrooms, the number one factor in the learning process is that students need to care and be curious. If they don't care, if there is no amount of curiosity then learning retention will not happen. I think this is why more students come to yoga following a health crisis or big life change. Many students come to yoga when they are pregnant because they take their wellbeing more seriously when it is connected to their baby's wellbeing. Most learning takes place when the brain is challenged to frustration, yet the task is achievable. Not over- or under-challenging is the key to material being learned. I would say that this is the same place we are looking for physically in a dynamic pose.

True learning, or understanding and mastery, is a process that takes both repeated practice and concentration. If you don't have students coming regularly to your sessions, then they will not be able to actually learn. Remembering this might help you to extend sympathy toward yourself and your students if you are mainly teaching drop-in classes that don't have a regular group of attendees. One of the reasons I love teaching courses, trainings and retreats is that I have a chance to see people actually learn in a clear way. Another reality of the yoga industry in big cities is the trend toward programs that offer major discounts through multiple studios, like *classpass* or *myclubs*, which offer students the ability to drop in on hundreds of different types of classes at different locations. Knowing that this culture of dropping in is a block to anyone's learning process helps me understand when students in certain studios don't progress. As a teacher I do my best to teach in an organized and inclusive way, no matter how long or short the time frame to teach is. An ideal situation is to see students regularly for learning to take place. If you are teaching in an environment that isn't supporting that, it might be time to think out of the box about how you offer your teaching.

Pro tip
Think about the trainings you have gone through and which model was really the most effective for your learning process. What are the models that you use, how long are your students in the learning process, when are the breaks and what tools do you use as a teacher? Would you be able to shift the way you teach toward a more effective educational model?

7

HOW WE TEACH

Authenticity comes from a balanced connection to your inner world and the outer world. Just like any relationship, staying in touch with your needs and the needs of another is a constant dance. When we teach, either individuals or groups, we are in relationship—to our students, our environment, our material and ourselves. Of course, the more practice we have, the easier this dance becomes. This chapter is about finding the practical tools as a teacher that will allow you to be authentic while also knowledgeable on techniques that enhance learning.

We know that one of the strongest factors in a learner's experience is the environment or atmosphere that they are educated in. Students who feel uncomfortable will learn less than students who do. If we are concerned for our safety and our defenses are up, we are not open to learning poses or being able to have a deeper experience of our yoga practice that goes beyond physical. It is important that we recognize and choose the type of atmosphere we create as teachers. In the yoga traditions certain styles and teachers are known for using harsh methods, for instance shaming students when they enter late or even using slaps and aggressive touch. I've heard stories of B.K.S. Iyengar slapping students. I've been in a room of over 60 students when a star level teacher yelled at one student. We have to be willing to look at the attitude that teachers bring to the class. Even when we admire someone's teaching for content or influence it is vital that we see the whole picture. Personally, I choose not to be in classes that promote shaming or unsafe touch. I want my students to feel empowered, so my attitude has to leave space for the students. Hierarchy is always part of group dynamics; however, I do my best to use non-violent communication (NVC) and promote questioning and openness. My way isn't the only way; it might not even be the best way but it is the best I have come to at this point in my journey. As the teacher I offer this to my students. I do not teach alignment as dogma, any more than I would philosophy. For me, creating an ambience that is friendly and safe is key in promoting learning. I find it sad that many teachers reach a level of notoriety and their egos seem to take over the room. That being said, to maintain respect for the group and the practice there are boundaries it is my job to uphold. Upholding those boundaries requires me to be assertive, to be an authority so that learning can take place.

Humility is a part of this role of teacher. I recognize that people have come to practice with me and that both humbles and honors me. If I want the quality of my teaching to be high, I need to acknowledge the quality within the room or structure that I am teaching. My students are equal to me and knowing this keeps me humble. I see my role as that of passing information, of guiding and shining light where there might have been shadow. Coming back to defining my role helps me to do it well. Another concept that helps me keep my boundaries and understand them is to remember that boundaries are not only walls for keeping separation. Boundaries are also the places of contact. Skin is a boundary, yet it is how we feel or contact the world. A boundary provides an opportunity for connection.

GOING INWARD: BOUNDARIES

What was a moment when you felt your boundary was crossed?

_____

_____

_____

_____

_____

What was a moment when you held your boundary well?

_____

_____

_____

_____

_____

What was the difference in both inner and outer scenarios between these two different examples?

_____

_____

_____

_____

_____

What helps you to uphold your boundaries?

_____

_____

_____

_____

_____

Name teachers that you admire that have clear boundaries.

_____

_____

_____

_____

_____

What are their qualities?

_____

_____

_____

_____

_____

ADJUST, ASSIST: JUST ASK

I used to start my classes by asking people to let me know about injuries and if they didn't want any hands-on adjustments. Some studios use little coin-like tokens that students can put in front of their mat to show whether they are for or against receiving hands-on adjustments that day. I have not worked with these and I have found that most students don't know about them even when they are there. The idea is great, and really helps bring a shift to the culture of teachers giving adjustments that might cross the line and are not done in a way that gives space for students to say no. Due to the prevalence of students being abused or injured through adjustments I use them less and less, as well as changing my approach. About seven years ago I started asking permission to touch in each moment before giving an adjustment. Then I started asking permission to touch each area of the body also. In a slow class like yin or restorative I find this last way most effective. In a class that is flow based it is not possible. For flow-based teaching I am even more concerned with finding other tools to teach with. This topic is very relevant and if we want to be able to continue using physical assisting or adjusting we must use even more care and sensitivity in doing so. In a workshop of around 100 other students led by another "international star teacher," when an assistant of hers aggressively adjusted me without asking permission or asking about injuries, my "no thank you" was barely acknowledged, partially because of the pace of the flow and partially due to the environment in the room. I consider myself lucky to have never been touched inappropriately or violated as so many students have been at the hands of yoga teachers. I do have injuries that are from strong adjustments from teachers who clearly thought they knew more about my body than I did. If we use physical contact as a teaching tool it has to be with consent, it has to be safe and guided by the student's body not from force. We also need to be willing to to tell our teachers no and to give feedback when something isn't right. Taking responsibility for moments we let someone manipulate our body in a way that was injurious is not easy. Saying no to someone who seems to know what they are doing is not easy. These actions are part of being a student, they are part of being empowered by your self-awareness, which ideally is a byproduct if not the essence of having a yoga practice.

Tactile teaching is great for learning. I do not want to dissuade teachers from using hands-on adjustments. I do know that it should be the last resort when teaching. In order to protect yourself and your students first communicate your instructions verbally. Next, use demonstration for the visual element. This can be done with another student's pose; it does not mean that you as the teacher need to do every pose that you want to show something about. Avoiding demonstration will help keep you safer if you are not warmed up and will help maintain your energy so that you are not overworking. The next approach is to have the students use their own hands, instead of you using yours. I will often instruct students in giving themselves adjustments, so that they can literally feel their own bodies. This is really effective. When I am adjusting a student, my main principle is that I want them to learn how to do it, so I will ask them to move a body part toward or away from my touch rather than me moving them. I avoid picking up my students' arms or legs. I am careful to assist their movement or actions with words at the same time as touch so they are informed and clear about how and why I am using touch. The clearer you are about how and why you touch, the safer your students will be and this teaching tool will become more effective.

Teaching method in order of safety and broadest reach:

1. verbal instructions

2. visual

3. tactile.

Keeping this order in mind will also help you in continuing to find your own words and more creative ways to teach.

TIMEKEEPING

Respecting time is a big boundary to hold as a teacher. I work to end my classes on time. When I don't have a clock in view, I can teach for hours without noticing the time. For me it is important to start and end on time. In drop-in classes it is important to know how late you will accept students. For me ten minutes is my limit for late students. I once had someone try to come in to a 90-minute class about 45 minutes late. It really shocked me (if you teach long enough you will see it all) and I turned him away. It was too disruptive for me to have him come in at that point, I didn't like the message it sent to the students that had come on time. The main issue in many weekly classes seems to be people who need to leave early. When people tell me before class that they need to leave early my request is that they go before savasana, or in a restorative class before the last pose. I offer to put their mat and props away for them and ask that they leave quietly while the rest of the students are setting up for rest. Most students appreciate this, yet on occasion there have been some who try to push me and insist on staying for the beginning of savasana. I really hold the line against this. It really disrupts the integrity of the group when one person has to walk through the quiet room. Barring an emergency, the end of the class is a sacred time for me to hold space so that the students can fully let go. When one student really insisted on staying longer, I had to use all my NVC skills to hold the line. It was not an easy moment. After the class another student who had overheard the conversation thanked me for sticking to my guns and she shared how difficult it is for her when people leave during savasana.

Leading trainings and retreats with long days can be another tricky point to keep the start and stop points clear. On first meeting a new group I explain that arriving on time is a way of respecting the work and each other. I outline the day so they know we get breaks and feel secure in the plan. The breaks are good for the learning process as they improve concentration. When I teach all day I am really strict about starting and ending on time, as much for myself as for the others!

INCLUSIVE LANGUAGE = SAFE LEARNING ENVIRONMENT

This is more than recognizing that pronouns should be used sensitively and LGBTQ, disabled people and students of all walks of life deserve to be welcomed in the yoga class. This is also more than understanding the cultural appropriation inherent in many Western yoga practices. As yoga becomes more common in Western culture, I think it is important to honor and respect the original Indian culture that yoga practice and philosophy began with. Inclusive language is about not assuming that your students have the same background as you, not judging them by their looks, and avoiding examples in your teaching that are not relatable to someone from a different socio-economic background. For example, I was in a workshop where the teacher was lamenting that there are not enough cleaning ladies as a way of explaining the feeling of being unsupported and overworked. I looked around the room wondering how many of the students in the room had cleaning ladies, or if anyone worked as a cleaner. As someone who didn't have a "cleaning lady" this reference completely left me cold and pushed me away from the teacher. I found it hard to learn for the rest of the workshop after this initial disconnect. Finding this kind of sensitivity is part of taking yoga out of the world of privilege and sharing it with people from different roots and worlds.

The next level of inclusive language is being careful not to tell people what to feel, but to leave enough space in what we say that everyone has room for their individual experience. We need to be sensitive to the fact that each pose creates different emotional and physical reactions in people. Just as we cannot assume the physical postures that challenge our bodies also challenge another, we cannot prescribe emotional texture to poses without alienating someone. I've been in classes before where teachers said simple things like, "Feel the pleasure of a deep breath," when in reality a deep breath is not pleasurable for everyone. If I'm in a strong emotional state maybe there is pain or physical discomfort in breathing deeply. Phrasing this differently would leave space for each individual to remain present and on another level to feel accepted by, for example, asking a question, "Is there any pleasure in taking a deep breath?" or making a statement, "As you take a deep breath, notice if there is pleasure in the process of breathing." Shifting your language in this way makes a massive difference to whether you are creating a truly inclusive class or prescribing your students' experience and assuming it is similar to yours.

PRACTICAL TEACHING SKILLS

One of the hardest things for newer teachers is giving instructions based on what the students need to do, which is responding to the moment instead of a script or fixed idea we have about what to say when. This is improvisation! Cues need to be given based on what you observe in the students. A big trap is giving cues that are unnecessary simply because you have heard them before. Keeping your eyes on the students instead of doing the poses yourself or closing your eyes will give you the information you need to know what to say.

Seeing your students will also help you know what to teach, not just cues but also what poses would be most beneficial for them. When they are struggling to get into a pose and you can imagine why, you have the freedom to teach something that will help them get there eventually. Understanding what is involved in each pose so that you can break elements down for students is key. Ideally, in any teacher training program you are learning about the key muscles and actions needed to build a pose. If this part of your education is lacking, please get some more training so that when you do see students struggle you are able to help them. Being well informed about cues comes from watching people react to what you say. If you repeat a cue that makes sense to you but no one is responding, clearly it isn't working and you need to find other words that do land. When I worked with a small group of trainee teachers they were very confused about the fact that not all cues work for all body types. The more you watch your students, the easier it will become to give cues that counterbalance so that in a large group the main tendencies are addressed.

Another challenge in many classes is teaching multiple levels at the same time. In the field of education this is called differentiation. This seems inevitable as there are no prerequisites for most yoga classes and a lot of students see themselves as intermediate after only two classes. Each pose we teach needs also to have a modification or option that will be accessible for someone at both a higher and lower skill level. In a flow-based class I have seen teachers call out, "Level one child's pose, level two downward dog, level three vinyasa." This can be a clear way to keep many levels content but it doesn't give much space for teaching people how to progress along the levels. I favor starting a flow-based class with a heavily modified vinyasa, then slowly progressing so that some students are able to integrate learning the vinyasa. At the same time, I always give options for balasana adho muhka svanasana as well as continuing to modify the vinyasa safely to make it easier or more challenging. Learning how to handle many levels is in effect teaching a sequence that offers basic learning blocks so that you keep all levels interested. One of the most commonly reported learning obstacles is that material is either too slow or too fast, usually too slow for half the room and too fast for the other half—so finding the right level is key to teaching well.

Considering the attention span of our students is also important, perhaps more so in longer sessions. Multi-screen and constantly distracting technology have shrunk the average attention span. They have also led many people to be more visually focused than before. When you are in a position to use PowerPoint slides and other visual aids, take the time to think about translating the information into verbal and kinesthetic or tactile forms. Is there something that can be passed around and touched instead of a slide to look at? One of my favorite teaching tools is using everyday objects—a French press coffee pot to show the movement of the diaphragm, the nozzle of a hairdryer in a tea mug to demonstrate the femur in the acetabulum. When teaching the functions of the body and kinesiology, the possibilities are endless. Check out children's science toys to get inspiration, and think back to when you were in school and how the teachers kept your interest in creative ways.

To optimize learning, we can also use the community model. Many people learn best working with others, not just in the same room. Partnering and doing group work is a fantastic way to keep everyone interested, sustain concentration and build sangha, or community. I love to use partner work in regular classes as a teaching tool, and I always give students the option not to work with another. I say something to the effect that, if you are not in the mood to work with someone else, and we all have those days, hang back and I will give you an alternative. It's important to me that no one feel forced to participate in partner work if it's a drop-in class and they are not expecting it or comfortable with it. In teacher training and longer workshops I use it more and also a lot of games that get the whole group on their feet or working in teams.

Here are some models and ideas to enhance your teaching:

Inquiry-based instruction

Creates high engagement—asking questions in ways that reach different people:

- Science-based—anatomy questions, physics!

- Subjective—philosophy, beliefs, "Do all triangle poses have to look like this?"

Cooperative and interactive learning

- Teamwork

- games

- diads

- puzzles/quizzes

- setting up stations for poses.

Visual aids

- PowerPoint

- objects (e.g. French press coffee pot)

- experiments

- demonstrations

- drawings

- skeletons

- muscles

- interactive white boards/flip charts

- slide shows

- tablets

- photos

- social media

- students video each other—create projects.

Compassion: the strongest tool

In Chapter 3 I mentioned a discussion with trainees on the 200-hour training about what we like or dislike in teachers. In this chapter I want to address some of the elements that are more enigmatic. They listed as positives: allowing personality and humor to come through, telling stories and weaving in philosophy. On the flip side, when asked what didn't work well these responses stood out: too much personal information or joking, strict or dry attitude, childish words and imagery that doesn't make sense or is vague.

Then the conversation turned to moments when teachers lose their cool and get into arguments with students. As much as we work to stay in contact with ourselves and be open to working with all types of people, we are human and we can all get triggered by students. The longer you teach, the more opportunities to get triggered will arise! Here we must circle back to our own practices that go beyond the physical, the inner work that is required to be self-aware and find healthy and supportive ways to express the inevitable emotions that come from working with people. Teaching yoga is very much a service job, one that requires us to be in close contact with people. One story of a teacher insisting on a student doing balasana (child's pose) in a different way led to a fight that disrupted the whole class. As most of us consider balasana a gentle and peaceful pose that is often used to rest, it might be difficult to imagine getting into an argument with a student about it. Since it is far-fetched to see it as a point of contention, let's use this pose as a jumping-off place for a compassion exercise. Beginning with something neutral is a good lead-in to working on building compassion.

GOING INWARD: FINDING COMPASSION

Imagine you are the teacher from the story above. What situation might trigger a strong emotional reaction to the way a student is doing balasana?

_____

_____

_____

_____

_____

What circumstances within you might be the kind of inner kindling that could fuel a fiery outburst?

_____

_____

_____

_____

_____

Are you able to have compassion for the teacher?

_____

_____

_____

_____

_____

Imagine you are the student. What situation might trigger a strong emotional reaction to the way a teacher is asking you to do balasana?

_____

_____

_____

_____

_____

What circumstances within you might be the kind of inner kindling that would fuel a fiery outburst?

_____

_____

_____

_____

_____

Are you able to have compassion for the student?

_____

_____

_____

_____

_____

I hope this exercise is one that can be applied to any conflict in order to bring some of the yogic philosophy from the *Yoga Sutras of Patanjali* into your daily teaching life. This exercise is based on my interpretation of Sutra 1.33:

> By cultivating attitudes of friendliness toward the happy, compassion for the unhappy, delight in the virtuous and disregard toward the wicked, the mind-stuff retains its undisturbed calmness.[16]

It is the second element in this list that applies most on this subject. To further explore this take some time to journal or ponder these questions:

When I am uncomfortable with my students' behavior am I able to stay calm?

_____

_____

_____

_____

_____

Am I able to see another's point of view, even if I do not agree with it?

_____

_____

_____

_____

_____

Am I able to stay connected with students and hold space for them even if they trigger me?

_____

_____

_____

_____

_____

Can I see how my inner reaction to students affects my attitude and ability to hold space?

_____

_____

_____

_____

_____

Am I self-aware when teaching?

_____

_____

_____

_____

_____

Am I able to have compassion for myself when I react or feel triggered?

_____

_____

_____

_____

_____

Who are the people I can talk to about difficult yoga teaching situations, or students that trigger me?

_____

_____

_____

_____

_____

Nonviolent communication

Learning nonviolent communication (NVC) is like learning a new language. I was first introduced to the technique during my time at Esalen Institute in 2006 and since then I have been thankful to have it as a tool. It takes a lot of work to speak this language and I am continually learning more. It is a technique that helps us to uncover our true intentions and own our feelings. Finding the words that describe feelings can be tricky as most of us actually articulate thoughts and ideas when we are trying to describe our emotions. The heart of this practice is finding a way to be heard by another and opening ourselves to seeing things from another's perspective.

These are the steps to follow:

1. *State an observation.* An observation must be a fact, not an opinion.

2. *Express your feelings.* This is where you might need to consult a list of feelings that are not causal, as in something that is only possible when someone else is involved. An example is the word "rejected." One can only feel rejected in relation to another. It inherently blames the other person for the feeling. More precise and autonomous feeling words include "lonely," "sad," "cold," "shocked," "hurt," "angry."

3. *State your need.* What is your deeper need, something that does not depend on one person, time or place? An example of a universal need is connection.

4. *Make a request for a clear action from the other.* This is something that works best when it is not a demand. If we ask for something to be given freely, it must be devoid of guilt or obligation. A request includes positive options and often needs time for us to consider what a genuine request would be.

It begins with using a script that reads something like:

When I observe [insert fact], I feel [insert feeling word] because my need for [insert need] is not met. Would you be willing to [insert request]?

A teaching example is:

> When I hear you asking to leave during savasana I feel uncomfortable because my need to create a safe atmosphere in this class during relaxation is not being met. Would you be willing to leave before we begin savasana in order to respect my needs and the class?

This is a brief summary and is only meant to introduce you to the concept. For further study I recommend starting with the brilliant book *What We Say Matters* by Judith Hanson Lasater and Ike K. Lasater. I also recommend checking out resource lists for understanding feeling words.[17]

8

PUTTING IT ALL TOGETHER

There is a difference between leading an exercise class and being a yoga teacher. I hope that this guidebook is helping you to clarify that for yourself as you define what you want your working definition of yoga teacher to be. If you want to have a long career as a teacher, strengthening your verbal teaching skills is a must. In the past when I have been injured or pregnant and unable to demonstrate poses myself, I was saved by the fact that my other teaching skills were strong enough. The shift from doing poses in front of the room, more like a leader of an exercise class, to seeing your students and teaching them in the moment will come from practice and doing the work set out in this book.

This chapter includes examples of teaching choices as well as some advice and sharing from colleagues of mine that I respect.

OPENING RITUALS

I want to bring us full circle, back to ourselves. At the beginning of this book I had you underline the importance of taking care of yourself to keep your voice strong. This goes beyond eating and sleeping; it involves self-honesty and the ability to feel your feelings. Whether you consider yourself an empath or not, teaching yoga is a very giving act and we expend a lot of energy when we teach. Building in a ritualized moment at the start of your teaching to have a self-check-in is a huge part of being present. I cannot tell you all the ways that recognizing how you are feeling, or simply noticing what is going on with an attitude of acceptance, will free up your energy and give you the ability to be present. It has been said many times before and I will say it again, repressing our shadow side only gives it power. The amount of effort required to push away any negative feeling or a feeling that you are judging as out of place when you go to teach is more than most of us can spare and be able to teach authentically at the same time.

Here's an example from someone who did my course and also worked with me privately. When we began with our vocal exercises, she seemed distracted, and during the practice teaching sessions she struggled with looking the others in the eye and with her volume. People couldn't hear her and her downcast eyes made her seem disengaged, as if she didn't want to be there. I coached her to stop and check in with how she was feeling and to share it if she was able. She said that she felt tired, and I coached her to say it a few times and each time to tell herself that it was OK to be tired. This took less than a minute. After she accepted that she was tired, instead of pretending she wasn't or judging it or telling herself that she shouldn't be, there was shift. When she started over, her voice was stronger and we could hear her more clearly. She had a power in her that was real and came across because she was no longer hiding. When she looked out at the people she was working with there was a connection and people began to smile. Then she began to smile. By acknowledging her truth and then applying herself to the task at hand she was able to do her best, to bring herself fully to what she did. It was a breakthrough for her.

We have to recognize that when we arrive to teach a class, we bring all of our baggage with us. We bring along the conversations from earlier in the day, the interactions during our journey to the class and whatever else our "monkey minds" have going on. Building into your teaching routine a moment for you to center yourself, check in and acknowledge your inner state will give you the ability to connect and do your job well. Whether this moment happens before you step into the room or during the time that you provide for your students to arrive and center is up to you. I know some teachers who sit and meditate in the room, so that while students are entering they are in meditation. I have seen teachers smudge the room with incense or light candles as they take deep breaths to arrive. For me the time that I use at the beginning of the class to guide my students in arriving and checking in is the time I am simultaneously checking in also. This is my time to remember why I am there. As I guide students to set an intention or san kalpa, I am finding my own intention in teaching and consciously noticing my inner state so that I am not using any energy to hide my feelings from myself. If I'm having a particularly emotional and challenging day, I might need to do some prānāyāma along with my students at the start of the class. Doing this while the class is in a comfortable or restorative pose with their eyes closed allows me to have a little more time to shift my focus toward the job. A few extra minutes for an opening can make the whole class much smoother.

I know some teachers who have special mantras they repeat before they begin. I say "how human of me" to myself after I notice my state. I breathe. Then I have the space to look at the people in the room and remember the reason I am there. This helps me to be present, not wearing the mask that hides my difficult feelings nor allowing them to be the focus.

Vocal warm-ups are best done before you teach. Even if it is only a few hums and a few face-stretching yawns, taking some time before you teach to warm up your voice is key to keeping it healthy and developing your vocal skills. At home in your practice the breathing and voicing exercises are meant to enhance your awareness and build healthy patterns. On the day you teach and need to use your voice you also need to warm it up! Take a few of the exercises that are most fun for you and create an opening warm-up that you can practice before you teach. It will make all the difference.

A lovely story from my teacher Judith is that she imagined her lineage of teachers standing behind her, so that when she began to teach she felt the connection to all of the teachers who had passed on their teaching to her. This was a spontaneous vision that came to her when she began her first class as a teacher. She continues to tell that story and I know many people benefit from remembering their own lineage when they need to feel supported.

GOING INWARD: HONORING LINEAGE

Take some time now to think of the yoga teachers who have passed their knowledge to you. Write down your lineage, or yoga heritage.

_____

_____

_____

_____

_____

List some ideas for your opening ritual.

_____

_____

_____

_____

CLOSING RITUALS

When I was teaching around 20 classes a week in London, I started to get headaches. I noticed a connection between these headaches and the classes I taught where I didn't feel a clear ending for my work. These were the classes that I would either rush off from or stay a really long time talking with students afterwards. I realized I needed a closing ritual, and a boundary for myself on how long to stay. When I was in massage school, I learned that I could use the time after a session to wash my hands not only physically but also to use cold water and energetically wash off the session. After I teach a class, I make it a point to wash my hands with cold water. Then I have a tea or a water and chat with anyone who has lingering questions. Or I give a hug to a student who is emotional.

When my drink is finished, I know that it's time to leave. It helps me immensely to have boundaries for myself, to have reminders to keep my wellbeing a priority.

GOING INWARD: CREATING CLOSURE

What are possible closing rituals that you can use?

_____

_____

_____

_____

_____

SHARING: HOW PERSONAL, HOW FUNNY?

Every teacher who has a following shares elements of their life in their teaching. This is what often reaches people more than a perfectly sequenced practice. As mentioned before, the amount of personal sharing and the context can either turn students on or off. So where is the line to be drawn? How do we lighten with jokes and not turn the class into our comedy show? Part of this will come with testing it out and asking for feedback. Another part will come from you working consistently enough to get a feel for it yourself. Here are some examples of times I felt teachers crossed the line into overshare or showing off.

In a vinyasa class with a strong ashtanga influence I attended in Vienna, the teacher was instructing the group through an opening meditation at the start of the class. Then he went up into handstand in the middle of the room. It had nothing to do with what he was saying; in fact, it was totally distracting considering we were supposed to be focusing inward. I found it bizarre and had a hard time letting go of my judgments throughout the whole class.

In a workshop at a friend's studio I gave an example of oversharing from a time when the teacher had apparently applied too much foot lotion and was slipping on her mat, and then she continued to talk about it for an extended amount of time. As I told this story my friend started to laugh because she had a similar story. Mentioning that your feet slip is one thing but going on and on about your foot lotion stops your students from being able to focus on their own feet. When you are sharing and adding anecdotes from your life, please ask yourself if it's relevant. The next story is from the opposite situation, a class where the teacher shared very little and did not allow her personality to be part of the teaching.

I know this teacher personally and for the last couple of years she has led group classes. From speaking with her I know she is passionate about yoga and serving people, as well as extremely knowledgeable when it comes to both yoga and functional movement through her training as a yoga therapist. From our discussion of anatomy, I was looking forward to her class. Unfortunately, it left me cold. I checked in with a friend who had been there also for her outside, non-yoga teacher perspective. She said it was "fine" but that she probably wouldn't go back. I think this is really common with drop-in classes: many teachers are not doing anything overtly "wrong" yet a lot of students don't feel the compulsion to return. Without breaking down the whole class, I want to explain why I think it didn't inspire, and show you how you can make sure that your classes reach the students who are open to your teaching so they will make it a point to come back.

A yoga class is like a story: it needs a good beginning, middle and end. One of the appeals of going to a yoga class is that it is a ritual. Whether you go for incense, candles and music or not, coming to a special place to practice yoga is ritual. All rituals and stories need a clear start. The class I went to did not have a start; the teacher didn't introduce herself or say hello. She did mention that she always has a plan and is also open to requests and any special needs. My friend asked for shoulder work. The teacher seemed happy to add shoulder and neck poses. Then she began the sequence, during which she mostly stayed on her own mat and did a lot of the poses along with us, sometimes modifying her poses but not explaining the options.

At certain points during different poses we were instructed to use three-part breathing, but that was never taught or fully defined. I wasn't sure if she meant viloma or some other way of breathing. The sequence is something I won't get into, but I will say there was a lack of middle—we didn't seem to warm up toward a peak pose or theme. Nor did we cool down for much time before savasana. During the sequence she repeatedly cued us to connect the hip to the leg, but there were no directional cues on how to actually do this, such as "scoop your hip under," "draw your sit bone back," "make sure the femur head is deep in the acetabulum" or any action that can be done to create the feeling of connecting the hip and leg. The practice seemed to be very focused on hips and included only few shoulder poses. At the end she announced that we had five minutes for savasana and she had some work to do on the desk so she would step outside, and that if people wanted to rest longer in savasana that was fine; however, she would let us know when the class ended in case anyone needed to leave on time. I found this very strange and the opposite of relaxing. She then stayed in the room and talked us through about a minute of instruction on keeping the mind focused on our inside if it wandered. After a few minutes she said that it was 11 o'clock, but that we could stay longer if we wanted. Then she left the room and went to the desk. There was no closing moment, no instruction on how to exit savasana, no namaste or thank you for coming.

It feels very critical to write out my experience of the class like this; however, I want to point out that I am not criticizing her as a person. She's a lovely person, yet her personality never came through in the class. Clearly, the focus on physical asana is prevalent in our current industry of yoga in the West. It is, however, important to remember that what makes any teacher stand out is their ability to inspire and encourage students. Inspiration comes through when you share yourself with your students through relatable stories that contribute to what you are teaching. It happens when you find ways to connect the physical movement to something deeper—not only heartfelt philosophy; even connecting it to the breath (which is still physical as opposed to spiritual) can elevate the student's experience. Thinking about the experience of the student as more than simply if and how to get them to do physical poses will shift your classes and help your teaching to become powerful. It is when our teaching has power, has a quality of human connection, that students prioritize making it to our classes and we begin to build a community and a career.

Every element of your class is a choice; whether you value teaching with Sanskrit, including philosophy or having a theme are elements that influence how the students feel in the class. Some students only want a physical approach; they might not care for any of the philosophy or have an interest in Sanskrit. I once had a student tell me after a class that he didn't want to know any of the "touchy-feely" stuff, to which I smiled and nodded. When I was a newer teacher, I took it very personally when someone had feedback for me that was less than glowing. Now I relish information that can help me improve how I teach, or even help me recognize who my students or audience really are. Someone who wants their yoga to be solely a workout without any mind–body–soul connection is not my target audience. Learning to be clear about what I do value in teaching yoga is a process that continues to help me grow as both a teacher and a yoga practitioner.

FROM THE TEACHER'S MAT

I wanted to include some stories from other yoga teachers to give you some different voices and perspectives.

Bridget Luff is a colleague of mine who was kind enough to write a short piece describing her personal ritual to connect with her authentic voice for yoga teaching. I hope you find it as touching as I did:

> I could be described as a fairly soft-spoken person. As a girl I was shy and felt uncomfortable speaking in class or in front of a group of people. Strangely though, I was able to get on a stage, inhabit a character and perform a part in front of a large audience. When I was more confident in the words that I was saying I was able to open up and channel a bigger truer voice within me.
>
> For those who are more softly spoken we are often told to "speak up" and it's not helpful to simply speak louder. It can make us feel more self-conscious and we strain to speak. It takes a lot of inner work to be able to modulate the voice and access that more primal part of ourselves that allows us to speak more freely. My pathway was through performance, which showed me that I didn't have to be just one type of person or have

one type of voice. Acting helped me step outside of the box of the "shy girl" and I learnt that I needed to give myself permission to step into my power.

This lesson was thankfully one that I was able to bring into teaching yoga. Although what was challenging for me at first as a yoga teacher was that I didn't get a script to learn or character to play. It's just me up there, sharing something deeply personal with people that I may have never met before and perhaps shall never meet again. I have found that sharing yoga takes deep courage and vulnerability, yet if I connect to what I am saying and why I am saying it then I am able to overcome my fear and find a strong clear voice that lies within me, that true voice that I believe we each possess.

To help me access my voice before teaching I always take a short moment (generally while I am setting up the room) to remember what really matters, why I have chosen to be a yoga teacher and what I hope to offer the people who are coming in. I set an intention for the class, whispering in my heart a short silent prayer. When I am connected to that deeper message my true voice can flow. As the class begins I try to make sure that I really see every person there, opening up to each of them. It's not always easy to do this as I feel quite naked and raw but I have found this to be the most rewarding way to teach. It's probably the only constant in my teaching—the setting of an intention and reminding myself of why I do what I do. Because if I lose that, I am flung back to being that mumbling little girl too shy to share the answer to the maths question, even though she knows it.

Adam Hocke is another London colleague that leads teacher trainings and co-teaches with Jason Crandell. He spoke to me about his view on common obstacles new teachers face as well as his process in becoming a teacher. This is from our interview:

> For me a turning point was to stop trying to be an entertainer. I came in full steam ahead with a lot of jokes and stories, trying to have charisma, which has its value and its place, but it turned into a bit of me wanting to be popular. What I needed to learn was how to use my performance experience in the service of keeping people engaged with what I had to teach, and not just try to make me the positive center of attention.
>
> I had a lot of helpful theater skills and tools from my background as a performer and playwright, especially not being afraid of talking in front of people, and knowing how to creatively present material and "sell" the content. But the continuing challenge has been not making it about me getting popularity or approval, which is hard because it is a big and competitive business.
>
> My advice to new teachers is to take the time to know what you are teaching, and then limit cues on a pose to no more than three or four at a time. Confidence and clarity come from limiting what you say and getting used to silence in the classroom. Don't be afraid to pause and breathe. Only start the instruction when you are ready!
>
> A pause that feels long to you is probably not noticeable to others and every teaching point can have a story and meaning connected to it. Let go of fear about using your own stories, let go of trying to be like your teacher. Focus on your own perspective and how to present that clearly in your own words. Make eye contact with students. Notice how you

feel when you are teaching and interacting with your students. Remember, it's not about you. After a "bad class," or a class when nothing went the way you thought it should, look back and remove your words and just think about the sequence. Did they do the poses? How would you feel if you did the poses? Remember that it's about how *your students* feel from the yoga. Have your own practices to support you and help you continue to teach.

Lizzie Lasater is an international teacher and the daughter of my own teacher Judith Hanson Lasater. Lizzie wrote this piece for my book, about how she found confidence in her journey as a yoga teacher:

I fell into teaching yoga.

It was 2005 and I was living in Los Angeles: studying Art History at UCLA in the mornings and practicing Mysore ashtanga with Maty Ezraty most afternoons. The summer before my last year at university, Maty announced she was selling YogaWorks, offering her last 200-hour teacher training and moving to Hawaii. Certain I was never going to become an actual yoga teacher, I nevertheless signed up for the training as a way to spend more time with Maty.

After the course I was surprised to get hired by YogaWorks and the UCLA gym to teach a few weekly classes. Feeling very much like an imposter, I didn't have a voice of my own when I taught. I'd stand at the front of the room and simply repeat the asana cues I'd memorized.

It was that feeling that turned me away from teaching yoga. I thought, how can I possibly make this into a fulfilling career? I don't even feel like I'm actually in the room while I'm teaching.

So I took a break. My life led me to design school in New York, and then to live in Europe with my Austrian husband. It was there, eight years after I stopped teaching yoga, that I began again. I was lonely and craving community. So I went to the local yoga studio and asked if I could teach restorative yoga. That first Thursday night class blossomed into my current path: offering workshops around the world and creating digital courses for yoga teachers.

Miraculously, this time around, I feel like I'm present in the room when I teach. I'm not exactly sure what's made the difference—perhaps it's life experience or a clearer sense of self. What I know is that I laugh more, and actually enjoy myself during class. I'm also able to see the students more clearly. It feels like it's more about them, and less about me.

David Kim is an international yoga teacher trainer and a senior teacher with YogaWorks. He wrote about finding his voice:

Before I started teaching yoga, I could not speak in front of a group of strangers without my heart feeling like it would burst out of my chest. According to some polls, the number one fear in America is public speaking (though clowns rank surprisingly high).

It wasn't asana that helped me overcome this social phobia, it was yoga philosophy. Practicing non-attachment to others' opinions about me meant overcoming my ego's distorted notion that people were constantly focused on what I was doing instead of their own nagging egos. In all of my trainings, I emphasize that yoga philosophy is as relevant now as it was thousands of years ago, except now we give it various names such as mindfulness, psychology, therapy, etc. So, one of the biggest highlights of completing a yoga teacher training is watching students boldly step into a space of vulnerability and wrestle their clingy egos in front of their fellow trainees. It may sound like they are teaching a pose but the underlying message is much more powerful: "I'm here now...deal with it."

9

EXPANDING AS A TEACHER

One image that comes to mind for many yoga teachers I know is that of a swan gliding on the water. The observer sees graceful movement and yet underneath there can be a frantic amount of legwork. When I began, I expected that at some point the frantic work underneath would lessen. After teaching for the last 16 (gulp) years I can tell you it does, but not all the time. If you are working steadily, different opportunities will arise and there will always be a growing edge. Now that I am leading trainings there is an immense amount of new administration and planning that has to happen behind the scenes, as well as more complex interpersonal situations with students. If you want to continue growing as a teacher, these different opportunities will help show you where your edges are and in what direction you want to go.

When I had my first interview with Elizabeth Stanley to work at The Life Centre she asked me who my teachers were. I think this is a brilliant question, which reveals whether a teacher is still learning. Continuing to learn and train is one of the most important things you can do for your teaching as well as for yourself. It will be the key to your expansion as a teacher. Finding a mentor is also a fabulous way to grow as a teacher. It is so rare that we have other teachers coming to our classes and offering honest feedback. Seek teachers that you respect and find mentors who will support you.

The most sustaining foundation that all longtime teachers need and have is a network of colleagues, a tribe. It is so important to find people to support you and continue to foster the relationships with friends who know the industry and are honest with you. Continuing to train is a great way to stay in touch with your tribe. Some of my favorite colleagues are people that I continue to study with, people to bounce ideas off and continue to learn with. Having a tribe makes all the difference.

Finding ways to keep filling your inspirational cup as well as taking good care of yourself will help you discover more work–life balance. When yoga begins as something that helps balance your life and then becomes your job, we sometimes need a different type of practice than only what we teach. This is why so many of the poses in Chapter 1 are restorative. I truly believe that resting and building your practice around finding a meditative state will enhance your teaching in a deep way. Creativity and the ideas that will make your teaching more an expressive art come from the quiet moments and the stillness that you create in order to listen to this silence. Another way to find silence and enter a deep meditative state is through yoga nidrā.

Yoga nidrā elicits the relaxation response while simultaneously shifting your awareness to something specific rather than simply the open silence of restorative yoga. Some people like to combine a nidrā practice with a restorative pose. I recommend you try it out for yourself and find what works best for you. Many think of yoga nidrā as a similar tool to self-hypnosis. Other people use it as a tool to help sleep or as a way to harness the power of the subconscious mind. My colleague and yoga nidrā specialist Thea Maillard kindly wrote the following nidrā practices specifically for this book. I hope you will enjoy them as much as I do.

YOGA NIDRĀ

Yoga nidrā is both a practice and a state of awareness. By doing a practice of yoga nidrā, we enter the territory of the state of awareness that is yoga nidrā.

Yoga nidrā is "a potent meditative resource for healing, insight, and empowerment."[18] It can be used for spiritual inquiries and development, for deep relaxation, creativity and problem solving.

Yoga nidrā is a safe practice for everyone. The yoga nidrās presented here are influenced and inspired by the work of my teachers Ben Wolff, Nirlipta Tuli and Uma Dinsmore-Tuli.

How to do this practice

The following script is intended for you to make your own yoga nidrā recording. For this purpose, you can read the script out loud and record it with a recording device or your phone. Reading from a script, however, is not how yoga nidrā is usually delivered. When yoga nidrā is delivered within the context of a class or workshop, the facilitator shares directly and authentically from their own experience of the practice and in response to the needs of the people in the room.

Please use the script only to make your own recording. If you are familiar with yoga nidrā and have a regular practice, you can share it with others, of course, but only if your sharing doesn't depend on reading from a script.

Before you record the nidrā, read the script out loud a few times to get familiar with the content. Yoga nidrā is a slow and meditative practice, so take your time reading the script, and make pauses where appropriate.

Preparation for yoga nidrā

You can practice yoga nidrā either lying down or sitting up in a comfortable position. The nervous system likes symmetry so aim to position your body evenly without crossing your ankles or legs.

Use any props such as bolsters, blankets, eye pillows and cushions to make sure that you are as comfortable as you'd like to be. Ensure that you are warm enough by putting on an extra layer or warm socks as your body temperature drops when you relax and remain still for some time. Turn off your phone and other devices for the duration of the yoga nidrā and, if possible, make sure that you are uninterrupted for the practice.

A practice for releasing nervous/anxious energy around teaching

Welcome to this practice of yoga nidrā.
And welcome home to yourself.
Allow yourself to be as comfortable as you'd like to be.
Do any adjustments to your body that help you settle into a place of comfort, wellbeing and deep rest.

Nidrā means sleep, and the idea for this practice is that the physical body becomes profoundly rested while the awareness is quite alert and attentive.

In the practice of yoga nidrā you need make no effort as there is nothing that needs to be done or achieved.

You are in the exact right place, at the exact right time.
Allow your body and your mind to settle.

The physical body settles into the loving embrace of mother Earth on every outbreath.
You are held and supported here.

And as the body settles, notice how the breath leaves the body all the way down to the bottom of the exhalation and how the breath enters the body all the way to the height of the inhalation.

Welcome the full cycle of each breath.

All the way down to the bottom of the exhalation, after the breath has gone all the way out.
And the all the way up to the heights of the inhalation, when the breath has come all the way in.

Welcome each cycle of each breath as if each breath were breathing you.

As if each cycle of breath contained within it a full cycle of a full day.

So as the breath comes in, that is like dawn arriving and sun rising.

And as the breath continues to rise all the way to the top of the inhale, that's like noon time, sun shining bright and full.

And then up and over into the afternoon of the breath when the air begins to leave and into the evening time of the breath and when all the breath has gone out, it's like being in the night time of the breath.

A quiet time. A time of waiting and rest.
Until the dawn of a new breath, when the next inhalation begins to arise again like the rising sun that moves from morning time to the height of noon and through the afternoon when the breath goes out into the night time when all the breath has gone out and there is nothing to do but wait until the next breath comes in.

And so on with every cycle of breath.

Noticing how the unfolding of the breath goes on and on and on.

And in that easeful rhythm of breath unfolding, the body settles deeper into stillness.

Now move your awareness to your heart space.

And then invite the whole body into this welcoming space of the heart.
Starting at the tip of the right-hand thumb, index finger, middle finger, ring finger and little finger.
Welcoming the whole of the right hand,
the back of the hand and the palm.
Welcoming the right wrist, forearm, elbow, upper arm, shoulder and arm pit.
Sending the welcome down the right side of the body through the ribcage and waist, down into the hip and buttocks.
The front of the right thigh and the back of the thigh.
Right knee, shin and calf.
Ankle, heel, top of the foot and sole.
Extending the welcome all the way into the right big toe, second toe, third toe, fourth toe and fifth toe.
The whole of the right side of the body welcomed into the loving energy of the heart space.

And then move the welcome into the tip of the left-hand thumb, index finger, middle finger, ring finger and little finger.
Welcoming the whole of the left hand,
the back of the hand and the palm.
Welcoming the left wrist, forearm, elbow, upper arm, shoulder and arm pit.
Sending the welcome down the left side of the body through the ribcage and waist, down into the hip and buttocks.
The front of the left thigh and the back of the thigh.
Left knee, shin and calf.

Ankle, heel, top of the foot and sole.
Extending the welcome all the way into the left big toe, second toe, third toe, fourth toe
*   and fifth toe.*
The whole of the left side of the body welcomed into the loving energy of the heart space.
The whole of the left side, the whole of the right side.

And then the welcome extends from the back of the heels up the calves,
back of knees,
hamstrings into the buttocks and lower back,
mid back, upper back and shoulders
into the neck and around the back of the head to the crown of the head.

Extending the welcome from the crown of the head to the third eye.
The little valley between the collar bones, the bottom of the throat.
Through the heart space.
Into the solar plexus.
The belly.
And all the way down to the bottom of the pelvis, the space of deep and inner knowing.

Welcoming the whole body, whole body, whole body.

And with every exhalation, feel the inside of your body, all the way down into the depth of
*   your experience.*
And with every inhalation, feel the outside of your body, the surface of your skin and the
*   space around you.*
Every exhale settles you more deeply into the depth of your body.
And with every inhalation feel the outside, the vastness of the space around your body.
Exhale—inside.
Inhale—outside.
Exhale—inside.
Inhale—outside.
The inner space. The outer space.

Now imagine yourself in a situation where you felt anxious or nervous about teaching or
*   speaking in front of a group of people.*
Imagine the situation represented by an image and hold that in the right hand.
Some people find it difficult to visualize
and if that is true for you, then find a word that represents the situation
and maybe you can imagine the word in big neon letters in your right hand.

And when you have that in your right hand, imagine for a second that you are living in
*   the world of opposites.*

And the opposite is true.

However you were,
you are now the opposite,
you are not like this at all.

And represent that with an image or word in your left hand.

Now there is either and or.

Now imagine having both the images at the eyebrow center, the Chidakash or Mind Space,
the black space behind the closed eyes.

It might be difficult or confusing to hold both images in the same place.
And for some people strange things happen here.
Maybe the images stay the same.
Maybe they change.

There is now either, or and both.

Now under the feet, where the feet touch the floor and there is no space,
perhaps between heel and floor,
there is nothingness.
Emptiness.
Void.

Imagining the sense of freedom that comes with the emptiness,
where there is no space between the foot and the floor,
where there is nothing between you and being grounded.

And when you have that sense, if you like,
you can copy that
as if copying and pasting it
from under the feet
and place that into the third eye, the Chidakash.
That nothingness
that freedom
that emptiness
the void
the space.

And when you have done that
copy and paste it to the right hand.
So now what's in the right hand is the same thing
that's in the third eye
and underneath the feet.
That void

that emptiness
that space
that freedom
the nothingness.

And if you wish
you can keep hold of the image in your left hand,
or you can replace it with
the freedom
and space
and emptiness
and nothingness.

And then take that space and freedom
and fill the whole body
from the tips of the toes to the crown of the head.
There is now no either, no or.
There is now no both.
There is now no neither.

And in this space allow your true self to be how your heart would like you to be.
Allow your true self to be able to do the things your heart would like you to do.
Allow yourself to feel the way your heart would like you to feel.
Allow yourself to look how your heart would like you to look.

And honor your heart by saying YES!

You can physically and mentally prepare now to come back to the body.

Take a deep breath all the way down to your pelvis.
And release.
The next breath goes into the depth of your belly.
And release.
Breath to your solar plexus.
And then to the heart center and maybe the body starts to wiggle and to move.
And when you breathe to your throat chakra you can release the breath with a little sigh
*   or hum.*
Breathe to your third eye and slowly open your eyes.
Come back into this room.

This practice of yoga nidrā is now complete.

A practice for vocal expression

Welcome to this practice of yoga nidrā.
Make yourself as comfortable as you would like to be
and know that while practicing yoga nidrā you can't do anything wrong
as there isn't anything that needs to be done.

Feel your body rest against the floor
and notice that you are held by the support from the floor beneath you.
Now draw your attention to your breath,
the natural flow of the breath entering and leaving the body.
Know that breath in the body flows in the same way
as water upon the Earth.

There need be no effort.
The breath lets itself in and out.
And if you observe an urge to control the breath,
see if you can let it go.
Just watch.

You can watch the breath in the same way you would watch waves
rolling in and out of the beach.

Let your breath be the guide into the state of awareness which is yoga nidrā.
In the rhythm of your breath
you can repeat to yourself:
I am practicing yoga nidrā
I am practicing yoga nidrā
Yoga nidrā is the form of practice.

Let your awareness now rest in the little valley
between your two collar bones.
Your fifth chakra
the space of creativity and vocal expression.

And if you like, imagine a blue light shining from the space
between your two collar bones.
If you find it difficult to imagine colors,
maybe you can sense or imagine a spaciousness at your fifth chakra.

And the blue light, or the spaciousness,
is now traveling through the body,
moving from the space between the collar bones
over into the right shoulder, and down the right arm
into the elbow, wrist.

Into the back of the hand and the palm
and then touching each finger in turn.
First the thumb, then the index finger, middle finger, ring finger and little finger,
so that the whole right arm and hand are filled
with blue light, with spaciousness.

And then the light fills the right armpit,
ribcage and waist,
traveling into the right hip, groin and buttocks.
Down the right thigh,
front and back.
Into the knee, chin and calf.
And into the heel, ankle,
top of the foot and sole
into the right big toe
second toe
third toe
fourth toe and fifth toe.

So that the whole right side of the body is filled with the spaciousness of the blue light.
Now move the awareness back to the space between the two collarbones
so that the light or spaciousness can fill the left side of the body as well,
starting at the left shoulder, and then down the left arm
into the elbow, wrist.
Into the back of the hand and the palm
and then touching each finger in turn.
First the thumb, then the index finger, middle finger, ring finger and little finger,
so that the whole left arm and hand are filled
with blue light, with spaciousness.

And then the light fills the left armpit,
ribcage and waist,
traveling into the left hip, groin and buttocks.
Down the left thigh,
front and back.
Into the knee, chin and calf.
And into the heel, ankle,
top of the foot and sole
into the left big toe
second toe
third toe
fourth toe and fifth toe.

So that the whole left side of the body is filled with the spaciousness of the blue light.
The left side and the whole right side.
And then let the spacious blue light travel up
from the heels
along the back of your legs
to your hips.
From the hips up the lower back
into the middle and upper back
into the neck and the back of your head.
And then up and over the crown of the head
into your forehead
and over the face
and the throat
into the chest
and down the front body
into the belly
and along the front of the thighs
and over the knees and shins
to the tops of the feet.
So now the whole body,
the left and the right side
the front and the back are filled with spaciousness.
The whole body.
Whole body.
Whole body.

And now bring the awareness back to your body
resting against the floor beneath you.
Feel the gentle pull of gravity holding your body against the floor.
With every exhalation let your body be heavy.
Grounded.
Held.
Like a rock.
And with every inhalation imagine the body to be light as a cloud.
Floating.
Free.

With every exhalation
the body is heavy as a rock.
With every inhalation the body becomes light as a cloud.
Exhale heavy.
Inhale light.

Exhale rock-like.
Inhale cloud-like.

And now see if you can feel both the heaviness and the lightness at the same time.
Like a floating rock.

And then simply let that go
and imagine something you would like to express in this world.
You can imagine it as a sound, a phrase, a smell, a picture...
Something that you would like to express or see happen
in your lifetime.
Something that the heart knows.
Take a second to listen to the heart and say YES!

This isn't about knowledge
because knowing won't get you very far.
This is about listening and loving and giving and being.

Take your expression to your heart and embody it within yourself.
It can simply be a sense
a feeling.

How would it be
to be a little bit more like that?
What would change?
How would it look?
How would it feel
and what would it be able to do?
What would that version of you wish to gift to the world?
Don't wait.
Be it NOW!
Your expression for the highest good of all concerned,
from a place of love.
From the heart,
to the heart.

And from this place of awareness,
which is yoga nidrā,
slowly bring yourself back to a more
everyday state of consciousness.

Let the breath be a little deeper and louder.
Wiggle the fingers and toes.
Yawn.

Stretch and move the body
in any way that feels comfortable to you right now.
Open your eyes.

This practice of yoga nidrā is now complete.

GETTING OUT THERE

As a teacher you are your own brand in terms of marketing and business. Finding your way within social media and marketing is part of the job of teaching yoga for most of us today. When I began teaching it was different—Facebook was just starting and there was no Instagram. Seeing social media as a medium for interaction and a tool for marketing will help make it something you play with and use rather than something that you measure yourself by. Find teachers that you admire for more than their number of followers and make sure that your feed helps feed your inspiration and imagination instead of only feeding the comparison that most of us fall into. Putting yourself out there online is similar to when you teach: stay true to what feels right and true to you. It gets easier the more you do it. Your perspective is what counts, not the reaction of people online.

Being prepared

Most teachers are paid for the time they spend preparing their classes. Not in the yoga industry. We do need to plan classes, and each of us will have a different style of planning. When I began, I would write out every pose and brainstorm themes that fit with the sequence. I also chose sequences based on physical asana that I wanted to get to or areas of the body I wanted to work on. Now I carefully plan workshops and trainings, but for drop-in classes I have a looser outline from which I can improvise. Sometimes I have a theme or peak pose I want to share, but it will always be possible for me to change my plan to fit the people. I see who comes to the room and that inspires what I teach that day. Some teachers use the same sequence all week long. Everyone is different. I encourage you to plan your classes taking into consideration the time of day as well as who will be there and the title of the class. I think about classes in terms of peaks and valleys, and whether I want to bring people's energy up for a morning session or to calm them down for an afternoon or evening session. These factors are important no matter what lineage or sequencing style I am working from.

Auditioning

Many studios will hold an audition class for you to start teaching there. This can be really nerve-racking, as being observed and judged is basically what an audition is. Be comfortable in your sequence. Allow for silence. Even when your students are the other teachers, give cues based on what you see and do the hands-on adjustments you would normally do. Treat them like any other group of students. If you are too nervous to interact with them, give a pose that allows you another moment to re-center. We all need child's pose. Don't be tempted to show your most advanced pose and make it about your ability to do a pose. Keep it simple so they can see how you teach and your personality. Do the work before to prepare yourself emotionally and mentally as laid out in the previous chapters.

Filming recorded practices

The internet provides a specific kind of platform for yoga teachers. From online sites that have paid memberships to YouTube and Instagram, you can self-produce videos from anywhere. Self-made videos have launched many yoga teachers into the spotlight and rocketed their careers; it's important to recognize the difference between being a yoga teacher and being a personality online or a spokesperson/model. Many people are a blend of these jobs, take a look at who you follow and in what way the mediums you choose to engage with actually work. I like the egalitarian aspect of sharing free videos, but I do hope that the teachers making the videos are clear about the marketing system they are participating in. It's important for us to know that those teachers offering free content to large followings are getting paid by marketing firms for the advertising that will come with that. This is also true of a lot of blogs and websites. Choosing your platform is important and it is also important when you work with any production company or online teaching platform that you have a contract and protect your creative material. Get a lawyer, know your rights and know what the company you are working with will provide.

When you go to film a video think of it like any class: who is your audience and what do you want to communicate? Remember that nerves are normal, don't let them trick your brain into thinking you are not prepared or capable! Find the time to relate to your feelings rather than repress them. Doing your vocal warm ups and having clear diction is even more important when the audience will be listening to you through a device. Many people have a feeling of stiffness or rigidity when they get in front of a camera. You can see this in a lot of videos when the teachers are not trained for camera work or used to it. Focus on movements and breath techniques that help loosen you up and work with people that help you to laugh when there is any technical issue (there always are technical issues). With any filming that has a crew expect delays, make time for a few takes and allow yourself to react as much as you can with your expressions and gestures. Use the warm ups from pages 72–6 to encourage a released and present body and mind. Facial expression on camera is going to have a big impact on the students. Like anything else, the more you do it the more comfortable you will get with it. Any feelings that seem amplified by the camera were probably there when you began teaching groups or did anything new. Going back to the exercises that guide you into a space of confidence are vital. Use the practices for relaxation from pages 167–176 combined with any of the restorative asana the day before you have a lot of filming or a big event.

Whenever possible, have a real student in the video with you to demonstrate and help your teaching. Do take care not to have your hand on the student throughout the practice, it looks like Thai-Yoga-Massage and can give the impression that the students watching the video are missing out! Know where the cameras are if there are multiple cameras, and when you speak to the camera imagine someone you find encouraging is standing behind it.

A great way to make your own videos is to separate the action and the sound. Start with your audio recording. Then play it back and follow the cues yourself to complete the film. Then cut it back together so that your voiceover goes with your visual teaching. This will help you to be clear about what you say and help you avoid speaking while in a pose. It takes more time but I think it's worthwhile whenever possible.

If you have online teachers that you enjoy or follow, look at how they work. Most teachers with a lot of followers have a whole production and marketing team behind their channels. It is the quality of your cueing that will make your recordings easy to follow or not. Essentialize what you want to say—cutting unnecessary chatter is even more important in a recording or any type of filmed class. Return to the language exercises on pages 96–100. Be easy on yourself as you find your own style and comfort level with teaching to the camera.

Utilize more tactile cues that are self-adjustments so that students have the benefit of their own physical touch. Try variations that encourage this, such as a twisting pose keeping a hand on the sacrum. Breathing practices with hands on the body are very helpful to counter the outward focus that can accompany looking at the screen for instruction. Use these hands-on cues to help keep your students in an embodied state, which can be harder for those who are not used to practicing in their own homes or with a screen instead of in person.

Livestreaming and interactive online classes

As I write this on April 29, 2020, most of the world is in a lockdown due to the COVID-19 pandemic. With the onset of regulations that have temporarily closed yoga studios and suspended public gatherings we have seen a rapid change in the yoga industry. Livestreaming or video conferencing has become the most common way of teaching. Many of us have been challenged as teachers not only to learn to use the technology, but also to deal with the emotional elements of growing again as teachers. Some feel as though they have to start over, particularly those who relied heavily on hands-on adjustments during their teaching and didn't develop the language skills to adequately describe detailed movement or actions. This process of shifting online has shown many of us where we need to grow as teachers.

The online options I'll examine are:

- interactive livestream classes

- non-interactive livestream classes

- online trainings/workshops/courses.

Interactive livestream classes

Interactive livestream requires conferencing software if you want to control the entry of participants. The main bonus is that you can see your students in real time, which gives you the opportunity to offer verbal adjustments and individualized instruction. This is only possible when you can see your students, which will require a larger screen for bigger groups so you can avoid scrolling. Some teachers use a projector, making sure it is a quiet one so the sound isn't a problem. Other teachers avoid demonstrating and simply sit close enough to their screen that they can see everyone. One option is to sit by the screen and spotlight the video of a dedicated student or assistant who has agreed to be the demonstration model throughout, so that you can focus on watching your students. Another option is of course going back and forth from your mat to demonstrate. Watching the students and giving feedback is very possible through this type of technology.

Livestreaming also offers a chance for students to have a check-in before or after class to provide some time for a community to build. This opportunity to see other people and connect through the screen has been invaluable to the mental health of many of my students: during this crisis some students are finding their only social interactions are happening before or after class. Having a group conversation on this kind of software requires us to wait until one person is done speaking before we begin. I like the slowing down of conversation and the way it invites us to truly listen for the pause in which to express our thoughts. It reminds me of the theater warm up where a group must count to 20 with only one person speaking at a time, any interruption or double talk sends you back to number one. This is a great game to play if you are having a longer discussion online, helping to break the ice and allow everyone to adjust to this form of interacting.

If you are concerned about creating an overly social atmosphere I suggest having clear boundaries about how you set up the class, perhaps stating on your website or when you email the link that you are opening the meeting for a set amount of time before and/or after the class. It's important to have a FAQs memo for those joining on how to deal with logging in and audio/video. You can also explain why it's important to have cameras on, and let people know that it's normal and OK for family or pets to walk through the room—basically to assure your students that real life is fine during the session. With all of us in our own homes and those spaces on display there is a more casual and possibly more intimate connection possible. Staying professional is still vital, however the lack of neutral space has the benefit of bringing a closeness, like a veil being lifted. I'm getting to know my students in a different way by seeing them in their own homes and they also get to know me by seeing my living room and hearing my family. Of course, in an ideal world we would have actual yoga props and more privacy from others in the house during practice, but the pandemic is teaching us to adapt and be ever more creative. I am finding this to be a beautiful though sometimes painful transformation for the art of teaching. I also think that students who used to struggle to have a home practice and depended on the environment of the yoga studio to create their practice space have an opportunity now to make yoga a part of daily life.

When the class officially begins make sure to turn the participants on mute so the sound quality of your microphone is better and there is less feedback or interference from other microphones. Staying sensitive to those in the group who don't want to share during a check-in or aren't comfortable having their camera on is part of creating an inclusive yoga room, even a virtual one.

Non-interactive livestream classes

This is most commonly done via social media—using IGTV, YouTube or Facebook you can "go live" and reach an audience for almost any length of time. Although you can't see your students, there are often lots of comments popping up at the bottom of the screen so move your screen to a place where it won't pull your focus. This platform is good for teaching a practice that you or someone else demonstrates throughout, with a fixed camera the entire time. It is most often used for donation-based or free content. The free content is usually either being compensated through advertising or the content itself is an advertisement for something more that will have a price attached. One more issue with these live platforms is that the anonymity of social media invites people to drop in and out, they might just pop over and look at what you are doing for a moment rather than actually practicing or learning. Facebook gives you the option to archive a live post, however Instagram only offers the live recording on your story for 24 hours. I wouldn't use this platform for deeper educational content.

Online trainings/workshops/courses

This form of education has been around for years, however with all yoga teacher trainings suspended at the moment it is becoming more popular; the Yoga Alliance are temporarily accepting 200- and 300-hour trainings done online. There are a lot of online trainings on how to make an online training! If you have a subject you want to cover more thoroughly and create a stream of income that does not require your time in the present moment, this format is worth investing in. There are websites like Thinkific or Udemy that provide you with the tools to create the material online and make it look professional, as well as giving you another place to advertise and find an audience. Yoga sites like YogaUonline, Yogacampus, Yoga Journal and Yoga International all offer different forms of online learning. There is a lot of creativity possible in this type of work, from scheduled live calls or webinars or forums for students to interact with you or with each other, to creating social media groups for each course. When planning a course the best advice I have heard so far is to be clear about exactly what you want to teach, and work backwards to create the lessons and curriculum to support the educational journey of your students. As most of us would never have imagined teaching a yoga class in person before experiencing any ourselves I think it is important to try different types of online learning to help you decide what you like, what supports your style of teaching and your content. There is so much to learn from noticing what you do and don't enjoy about these options.

Recordings of livestream classes

Always check privacy issues related to sharing any content that includes images of your students. I'm not a fan of seeing pictures where students are being used to market something when they are clearly just there to do a class. If you want to use any image that includes a student, for social media or your website or for educational purposes, you must get their written permission.

An easy way to build up your online offerings or compile something into a course is to use either video or audio from the live classes. Test out your recording equipment and start! You can offer these recordings as a passive stream of income.

Microphones

When you film professionally or teach a very large group you will most likely have a microphone. Get comfortable with any microphone that is placed on your clothes, test out the poses you will do and get the microphone secure and out of your way. Test your voice and find the sound person to see if your levels are good. Microphones pick up every little breath and spit sound, so this is where your diction work will really help you. When using a microphone, it can blast too loud or give feedback when your volume rises; this happens a lot if you are in a conference or large group. Work to keep your voice at more of an even volume, and if you want to get your voice booming on energetic moments, maybe you don't need the microphone!

LAST WORDS

It always helps me to remember that there is a lot going on underneath the surface of each human being, most of which I am often unaware of, even in myself. As animals we are built to constantly evaluate information from our environment and those around us to keep us safe. I am gleaning information from people, and vice versa, in every moment through the nervous system. In yoga philosophy we think of the human body as having layers like an onion. These layers are called *koshas* in Sanskrit. In moments when I am challenged by communication or the seeming lack thereof, I consider the many elements at play and remind myself that humans are complex and layered beings. This re-inspires my curiosity about the human experience, which is the passion that drives both my teaching and my practice. I hope this book will help you to explore your teaching practice with respect for your process and your students.

Notes

1   Seattle Yoga News (2019) *Yoga in America 2016*. Accessed December 17, 2019 at http://seattleyoganews.com/yoga-in-america-2016-statistics

2   Brown (2009) *Play: How It Shapes the Brain, Opens the Imagination, and Invigorates the Soul*. New York: Penguin Group.

3   Kuchera, M. (1997) 'Treatment of Gravitational Strain.' In A. Vleeming (ed.) *Movement, Stability, and Low Back Pain*. New York: Churchill Livingstone, p.17.

4   Desikachar, T.K.V. (1995) *The Heart of Yoga: Developing a Personal Practice*. Rochester, VT: Inner Traditions International, p.60.

5   Ashley-Farrand, T. (2003) *Shakti Mantras: Tapping into the Great Goddess Energy Within*. New York: Random House, p.33.

6   Satchidananda, Sri Swami (2012) *The Yoga Sutras of Patanjali*. Buckingham, VA: Integral Yoga Publications.

7   Linklater, K. (n.d.) 'The art and craft of voice (and speech) training. Experiential perspectives: reflections on voice and speech training.' Accessed on December 19, 2019 at www.linklatervoice.com/resources/articles-essays/42-the-art-and-craft-of-voice-and-speech-training#edn8

8   Created by Wilhelm Reich.

9   Morgan, M.K. (2012) *Constructing the Holistic Actor: Fitzmaurice Voicework©*. Scotts Valley, CA: Createspace Independent Publishing Platform, p.54.

10 Anderson, V.A. (1997) *Training the Speaking Voice* (3rd edition). New York: Oxford University Press. Reproduced with permission of Oxford Publishing Limited through PLSclear.

11 Johnstone, K. (2007) *Impro: Improvisation and the Theatre*. London: Bloomsbury, p.80.

12 Napier, M. (2004) *Improvise: Scene from the Inside Out*. Portsmouth, NH: Heinemann Drama, p.118.

13 Accessed on December 20, 2019 at Dictionary.com, www.dictionary.com/browse/body-language?s=t

14 Scientific American (2008) 'The mirror neuron revolution: explaining what makes humans social.' Accessed on December 20, 2019 at www.scientificamerican.com/article/the-mirror-neuron-revolut

15 Moreno, N., Miller, L., Tharp, B., Taber, K., Kabnick, K. and Dresden, J. (2016) *BrainLink The Motor System Teacher's Guide: BioEd Teacher Resources*. Houston, TX: Center for Educational Outreach, Baylor College of Medicine, p.1.

16 Satchidananda, Sri Swami (2012) *The Yoga Sutras of Patanjali*. Buckingham, VA: Integral Yoga Publications, p.51.

17 See, for example, New York Center for Nonviolent Communication (n.d.) *Feelings*, accessed on December 21, 2019 at www.nycnvc.org/feelings

18 Yoga Nidra Network (n.d.) *About the Yoga Nidra Network...* Accessed on December 20, 2019 at www.yoganidranetwork.org

Index